# Emerging Technologies in Thoracic Surgery

*Editor*

MICHAEL J. WEYANT

# THORACIC SURGERY CLINICS

www.thoracic.theclinics.com

*Consulting Editor*
VIRGINIA R. LITLE

August 2023 • Volume 33 • Number 3

**ELSEVIER**

1600 John F. Kennedy Boulevard • Suite 1800 • Philadelphia, Pennsylvania, 19103-2899

http://www.thoracic.theclinics.com

**THORACIC SURGERY CLINICS Volume 33, Number 3**
**August 2023 ISSN 1547-4127, ISBN-13: 978-0-443-18274-7**

**Editor:** John Vassallo (j.vassallo@elsevier.com)
**Developmental Editor:** Jessica Nicole B. Cañaberal



*Thoracic Surgery Clinics* (ISSN 1547-4127) is published quarterly by Elsevier Inc., 360 Park Avenue South, New York, NY 10010-1710. Months of publication are February, May, August, and November. Business and editorial offices: 1600 John F. Kennedy Boulevard, Suite 1800, Philadelphia, PA 19103-2899. Periodicals postage paid at New York, NY, and additional mailing offices. Subscription prices are $417.00 per year (US individuals), $681.00 per year (US institutions), $100.00 per year (US students), $487.00 per year (Canadian individuals), $881.00 per year (Canadian institutions), $100.00 per year (Canadian students), $225.00 per year (international students), $509.00 per year (international individuals), and $881.00 per year (international institutions). Foreign air speed delivery is included in all Clinics' subscription prices. All prices are subject to change without notice. **POSTMASTER:** Send address changes to Thoracic Surgery Clinics, Elsevier Health Sciences Division, Subscription Customer Service, 3251 Riverport Lane, Maryland Heights, MO 63043. **Customer Service (orders, claims, online, change of address): Telephone: 1-800-654-2452 (U.S. and Canada); 314-447-8871 (outside U.S. and Canada). Fax: 314-447-8029. E-mail: journalscustomerservice-usa@elsevier.com (for print support); journalsonlinesupport-usa@elsevier.com (for online support).**

*Reprints.* For copies of 100 or more, of articles in this publication, please contact Commercial Rights Department, Elsevier Inc., 360 Park Avenue South, New York, NY 10010-1710. Tel: 212-633-3874; Fax: 212-633-3820; E-mail: reprints@elsevier.com.

*Thoracic Surgery Clinics* is covered in *MEDLINE/PubMed (Index Medicus), EMBASE/Excerpta Medica, Science Citation Index Expanded (SciSearch®), Journal Citation Reports/Science Edition,* and *Current Contents®/Clinical Medicine.*

# Contributors

## CONSULTING EDITOR

**VIRGINIA R. LITLE, MD**
Chief of Thoracic Surgery, St. Elizabeth's Medical Center, Cambridge, Massachusetts, USA

## EDITOR

**MICHAEL J. WEYANT, MD**
Director, Inova Thoracic Surgery Program, Moran Family Endowed Chair in Thoracic Oncology, Professor, University of Virginia School of Medicine, Co-Director, Thoracic Oncology Program, Inova Schar Cancer Institute, Fairfax, Virginia, USA

## AUTHORS

**MAHWISH BARI, BS**
Clinical Research Coordinator, Lung/Interventional Pulmonology, Inova Schar Cancer Institute, Fairfax, Virginia, USA

**ANDREA BILLE, MD, PhD**
Department of Thoracic Surgery, Guy's and St Thomas' NHS Foundation Trust, Guy's Hospital, School of Cancer and Pharmaceutical Sciences, King's College London, London, United Kingdom

**BRYAN M. BURT, MD, FACS**
Division of Thoracic Surgery, The Michael E. Debakey Department of Surgery, Baylor College of Medicine, Houston, Texas, USA

**SHOURJO CHAKRAVORTY, MD**
Department of Medicine, Inova Fairfax Medical Center, Fairfax, Virginia, USA

**DUY KEVIN DUONG, MD, DAABIP**
Department of Interventional Pulmonology, Inova Schar Cancer Institute, Inova Fairfax Hospital, Fairfax, Virginia, USA

**MATTHEW R.L. EGYUD, MD**
Division of Thoracic Surgery, The Michael E. Debakey Department of Surgery, Baylor College of Medicine, Houston, Texas, USA

**KATHLEEN M.I. FUENTES, MD**
Department of General Surgery, Lahey Hospital and Medical Center, Burlington, Massachusetts, USA

**SIDHU P. GANGADHARAN, MD, MHCM**
Chief, Division of Thoracic Surgery and Interventional Pulmonology, Beth Israel Deaconess Medical Center, Associate Professor of Surgery, Harvard Medical School, Boston, Massachusetts, USA

**SCOTT HOLMES, CMI**
The Michael E. Debakey Department of Surgery, Baylor College of Medicine, Houston, Texas, USA

**TARYNE A. IMAI, MD, MEHP**
Director of Thoracic Surgery, The Queen's University Medical Group, Queen's Health System, University of Hawaii, Honolulu, Hawaii, USA

**BINIAM KIDANE, MD**
Department of Surgery, University of Manitoba, Winnipeg, Manitoba, Canada

**SAVVAS LAMPRIDIS, MD**
Guy's and St Thomas' NHS Foundation Trust, Department of Cardiothoracic Surgery,

Hammersmith Hospital, Imperial College Healthcare NHS Trust, London, United Kingdom

**NATALIE S. LUI, MD, MAS**
Assistant Professor, Department of Cardiothoracic Surgery, Stanford University School of Medicine, Stanford, California, USA

**AMIT K. MAHAJAN, MD, FCCP, DAABIP**
Medical Director, Interventional Pulmonologist, Inova Health System, Inova Schar Cancer Institute, Fairfax, Virginia, USA

**FLEMING MATHEW, MBBS**
Research Fellow, Division of Thoracic Surgery and Interventional Pulmonology, Beth Israel Deaconess Medical Center, Harvard Medical School, Boston, Massachusetts, USA

**PHILICIA MOONSAMY, MD, MPH**
Division of Thoracic Surgery, Massachusetts General Hospital, Boston, Massachusetts, USA

**KALPAJ R. PAREKH, MBBS**
Professor and Chair, Department of Cardiothoracic Surgery, University of Iowa Hospitals and Clinics, Iowa City, Iowa, USA

**BERNARD PARK, MD, FACS**
Attending Thoracic Surgeon, Division of Thoracic Surgery, Memorial Sloan Kettering Cancer Center, New York, New York, USA

**JU AE PARK, MD**
Department of General Surgery, Resident, Inova Fairfax Medical Campus, Fairfax, Virginia, USA

**PRIYA P. PATEL, MD, DAABIP**
Department of Interventional Pulmonology, Inova Schar Cancer Institute, Inova Fairfax Hospital, Fairfax, Virginia, USA

**ANTONIA A. PONTIKI, BEng**
School of Biomedical Engineering and Imaging Sciences, King's College London, Department of Surgical and Interventional Engineering, School of Biomedical Engineering and Imaging Sciences, The Rayne Institute, St Thomas' Hospital, London, United Kingdom

**KAWAL RHODE, PhD**
School of Biomedical Engineering and Imaging Sciences, King's College London, Department of Surgical and Interventional Engineering, School of Biomedical Engineering and Imaging Sciences, The Rayne Institute, St Thomas' Hospital, London, United Kingdom

**KENNETH P. SEASTEDT, MD**
Department of Surgery, Beth Israel Deaconess Medical Center, Harvard Medical School, Boston, Massachusetts, USA

**ELLIOT L. SERVAIS, MD**
Division of Thoracic Surgery, Lahey Hospital and Medical Center, Burlington, Massachusetts, USA

**KEI SUZUKI, MD, MS**
Inova Thoracic Surgery, Director of Thoracic Surgery Research, Inova Schar Cancer Institute, Fairfax, Virginia, USA

**ANTHONY M. SWATEK, MD**
Assistant Professor, Department of Cardiothoracic Surgery, University of Iowa Hospitals and Clinics, Iowa City, Iowa, USA

**LYE-YENG WONG, MD**
Resident Physician, Department of Cardiothoracic Surgery, Stanford University School of Medicine, Stanford, California, USA

# Contents

valves into segmental or subsegmental airways can induce lobar atelectasis for portions of diseased lung. This results in the reduction of hyperinflation along with improvements in diaphragmatic curvature and excursion.

**Advanced Endoscopy for Thoracic Surgeons** **251**

Kathleen M.I. Fuentes, Kenneth P. Seastedt, Biniam Kidane, and Elliot L. Servais

Video content accompanies this article at http://www.thoracic.theclinics.com.

The thoracic surgeon, well versed in advanced endoscopy, has an array of therapeutic options for foregut pathologic conditions. Peroral endoscopic myotomy (POEM) offers a less-invasive means to treat achalasia, and the authors' preferred approach is described in this article. They also describe variations of POEM, such as G-POEM, Z-POEM, and D-POEM. In addition, endoscopic stenting, endoluminal vacuum therapy, endoscopic internal drainage, and endoscopic suturing/clipping are discussed and can be valuable tools for esophageal leaks and perforations. Endoscopic procedures are advancing rapidly, and thoracic surgeons must maintain at the forefront of these technologies.

**Technical Aspects of Robotic First Rib Resection** **265**

Matthew R.L. Egyud, Scott Holmes, and Bryan M. Burt

Robot-assisted thoracoscopic surgery for the treatment of thoracic outlet syndrome is a novel approach that continues to increase in popularity due to advantages compared with traditional open first rib resection. Following publication of the Society of Vascular Surgeons expert statement in 2016, the diagnosis and management of thoracic outlet syndrome is favorably evolving. Technical mastery of the operation requires precise knowledge of anatomy, comfort with robotic surgical platforms, and understanding of the disease.

**Three-Dimensional Printing Applications in Thoracic Surgery** **273**

Antonia A. Pontiki, Kawal Rhode, Savvas Lampridis, and Andrea Bille

Advances in technology allowing the combination of medical imaging and three-dimensional printing have greatly benefitted thoracic surgery, allowing for the creation of complex prostheses. Surgical education is also a significant application of three-dimensional printing, especially for the development of simulation-based training models. Aiming to show how three-dimensional printing can benefit patients and clinicians in thoracic surgery, an optimized method to create patient-specific chest wall prosthesis using three-dimensional printing was developed and clinically validated. An artificial chest simulator for surgical training was also developed, replicating the human anatomy with high realism and accurately simulating a minimally invasive lobectomy.

**Uniportal Robotic Lung Resection Techniques** **283**

Philicia Moonsamy and Bernard Park

Uniportal video-assisted thoracic surgical (U-VATS) and telerobotic techniques have become widely adopted strategies for lung resection and represent a natural progression born of advancing technologic innovation and decades of expanding clinical experience. Combining the best that each approach offers may be the next logical step in the evolution of minimally invasive thoracic surgery. Two parallel efforts are underway: one that combines the traditional U-VATS incision with a multi-arm telerobotic platform and one that utilizes a new single-arm device. Feasibility and refinement of surgical technique will need to be achieved before any conclusions about efficacy can be drawn.

**Lung Xenotransplantation** 291

Anthony M. Swatek and Kalpaj R. Parekh

Although efforts have been made to expand the pool of donor lung allografts for human lung transplantation, a shortage remains. Lung xenotransplantation has been proposed as an alternative approach, but lung xenotransplantation in humans has not yet been reported. In addition, significant biological and ethical barriers will have to be addressed before clinical trials can be undertaken. However, significant progress has been made toward addressing biological incompatibilities that present a barrier, and recent advances in genetic engineering tools promise to accelerate further progress.

**Thermoablative Techniques to Treat Excessive Central Airway Collapse** 299

Sidhu P. Gangadharan and Fleming Mathew

Excessive central airway collapse (ECAC) is a condition characterized by the excessive narrowing of the trachea and mainstem bronchi during expiration, which can be caused by Tracheobronchomalacia (TBM) or Excessive Dynamic Airway Collapse (EDAC). The initial standard of care for central airway collapse is to address any underlying conditions such as asthma, COPD, and gastro-esophageal reflux. In severe cases, when medical treatment fails, a stent-trial is offered to determine if surgical correction is a viable option, and tracheobronchoplasty is suggested as a definitive treatment approach. Thermoablative bronchoscopic treatments, such as Argon plasma coagulation (APC) and laser techniques (potassium-titanyl-phosphate [KTP], holmium and yttrium aluminum pevroskyte [YAP]) are a promising alternative to traditional surgery. However, further research is needed to assess their safety and effectiveness in humans before being widely used.

# THORACIC SURGERY CLINICS

## FORTHCOMING ISSUES

***November 2023***
**Access to Lung Cancer Screening**
DuyKhanh P. Ceppa and Kei Suzuki, *Editors*

***February 2024***
**The Professional Lifespan: From Residency to Retirement**
Stephen C. Yang and Jinny S. Ha, *Editors*

***May 2024***
**Surgical Conditions of the Diaphragm**
Erin Alexis Gillaspie, *Editor*

## RECENT ISSUES

***May 2023***
**Controversies in Thoracic Surgery**
Lana Y. Schumacher and David C. Griffin, *Editors*

***February 2023***
**Robotic Thoracic Surgery**
Elliot L. Servais and Peter J. Smit, *Editors*

***November 2022***
**Esophageal Cancer**
Jonathan Yeung and Elena Elimova, *Editors*

# Foreword

# Calling All Budding Innovators and Surgeon Scientists to Thoracic Surgery

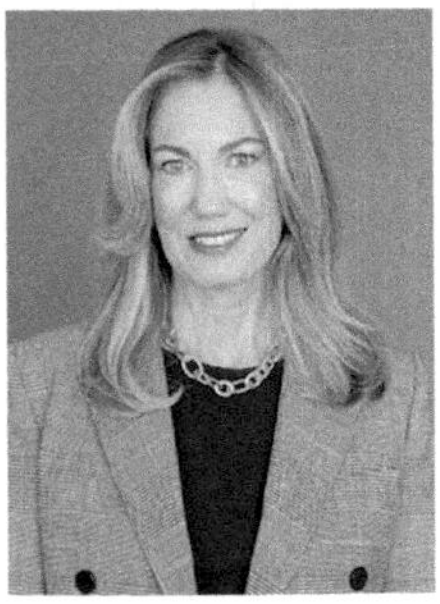

Virginia R. Litle, MD
*Consulting Editor*

Innovators and surgeon scientists: where would we be without those thought leaders in surgery? The excitement of hearing surgical innovators share their experiences should be infectious. At the 2023 American Surgical Association, President Diana Farmer, UC Davis Chair of Surgery, presented the path to her landmark Management of Myelomeningocele Study (MOMS) trial of prenatal versus postnatal repair of spina bifida. On the April 2023 episode of Society of Thoracic Surgeons "Same Surgeon, Different Light" podcast, Dr Bartley Griffith, University of Maryland Distinguished Professor of Surgery, discussed his first successful xenotransplantation of a genetically modified heart. Dr Yolonda Colson, the first woman President of American Association for Thoracic Surgery (AATS), has applied her surgeon-scientist skillset to advance the area of nanotechnology and intraoperative molecular imaging and subsequently mentored and inspired many young surgeons. These are just recently shared experiences reflecting innovative ideas, decades of exploration and development, and teamwork.

In this issue of *Thoracic Surgery Clinics*, Dr Michael Weyant has selected ten progressive and emerging topics in Thoracic Surgery, which encompass techniques, surgical approaches, and biomarker development for the broad field of thoracic surgery. For lung cancer, Park and Suzuki report novel screening tools for this still dreaded malignancy, and Wong and Lui summarize advances in intraoperative localization of malignant nodules. For benign airway pathology like excessive central airway collapse, Gangadharan and Mathew outline developing thermoablative techniques as an option over tracheobronchoplasty for some patients. We learn from Swateck and Parekh that lung xenotransplantation is still on the horizon, but that there is much fodder for basic science investigation in this arena. The role of three-dimensional printing in thoracic continues to expand in the area of surgical education and preoperative planning, but the use of readily available organ implants may not be too far off. This is just some of the content of this issue of *Thoracic Surgery Clinics*. Aside from the goal of presenting new and exciting topics, this issue should inspire Thoracic trainees and newly minted surgeons to get energized about what floats their boat: technical advances, esophageal pathology, chest

Thorac Surg Clin 33 (2023) ix–x
https://doi.org/10.1016/j.thorsurg.2023.05.002
1547-4127/23/© 2023 Published by Elsevier Inc.

wall problems, or benign and malignant lung disease? From hearing about the accomplishments of surgical leaders in-print, in-person, or on-podcast, young thoracic surgeons can appreciate the joy of creating your hypothesis, focusing on the methods, and finding your niche to benefit the patients and the field.

Thank you to Dr Weyant and to all the contributors of this issue about Emerging Technologies. May history repeat itself with producing successful surgeon scientists, but may the future be bright with surgical advances.

Virginia R. Litle, MD
St. Elizabeth's Medical Center
11 Nevins Street, Suite 20
Brighton, MA 02135 USA

*E-mail address:*
vlitle@gmail.com

# Preface
# Emerging Technologies in Thoracic Surgery

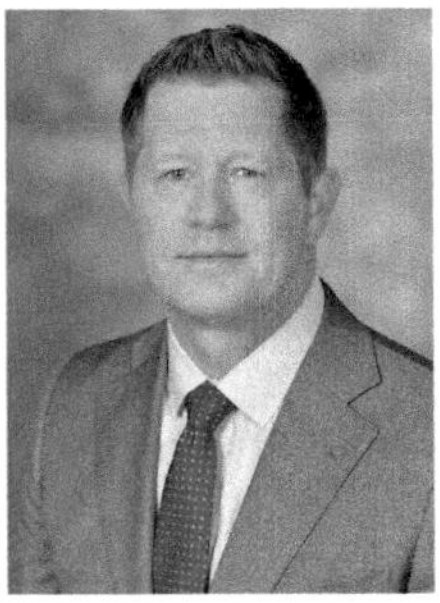

Michael J. Weyant, MD
*Editor*

The evolution of our practice as thoracic surgeons continues to lean toward more minimally invasive and endoscopic procedures. During the last decade, we have witnessed a transition from video-assisted thoracic surgical approaches to a robotic platform. This has been the source of much of the discussion at our specialty meetings and congresses. This revolution into robotic surgery has forced many surgeons to adopt an entirely new way of operating. Although sometimes difficult, transition to this platform has allowed more patients access to minimally invasive procedures to treat some of the most common diseases we see, namely lung cancer.[1,2]

This introduction of the robotic platform has been led by surgeons, and the training in these techniques has been disseminated by surgeons to surgeons. The decades in front of us will see the evolution of many more minimally invasive types of treatments, namely endoluminal therapies. The development of these technologies represents a unique dilemma for thoracic surgeons in that many of these new technologies are developed in other specialties, such as gastroenterology or interventional pulmonology. It makes sense, of course, that as medicine and surgery evolve, the types of treatment we provide will only get more minimally invasive, and this requires the willingness and ability to collaborate with specialists who are not technically trained as surgeons but rather as advanced proceduralists. For this reason, a significant portion of this issue is focused on topics that we currently collaborated in with our pulmonary and gastrointestinal colleagues.

As we all have observed, there is a growing number of thoracic surgery programs that are evolving into thoracic procedural service lines in which interventional pulmonologists and thoracic surgeons are housed in the same division or department. I have observed this directly, and I believe this type of noncompetitive collegial environment is the way of the future and will allow for more rapid and unbiased development of minimally invasive technology to treat our patients. These multidisciplinary efforts will also allow thoracic surgeons to be trained in all areas of minimally invasive pulmonary therapeutics in the future. This paradigm may also influence our interactions with our gastroenterology colleagues.

The remainder of this issue focuses on theoretical advances that we may witness, including lung transplantation using xenografts, intraoperative molecular imaging of tumors, and the potential use of three-dimensional printing in our specialty that may or may not become part of our clinical practice.

To provide a review of some of the latest advances in thoracic surgery, experts from multiple disciplines and geographic areas were invited to contribute their knowledge of specific areas of the latest developments in thoracic surgery as well as potential technology of the future. Although there is not a specific clinical theme for this issue, the topics represented touch on many areas that

Thorac Surg Clin 33 (2023) xi–xii
https://doi.org/10.1016/j.thorsurg.2023.05.001
1547-4127/23/© 2023 Published by Elsevier Inc.

are currently at the forefront of clinical practice and research in thoracic surgery. It has been a privilege to serve as an editor for this issue of *Thoracic Surgery Clinics* and to highlight some of the work being done by our colleagues.

Michael J. Weyant, MD
University of Virginia School of Medicine
INOVA Schar Cancer Institute
8081 Innovation Park Drive
Fairfax, VA 22031, USA

*E-mail address:*
michael.weyant@inova.org

## REFERENCES

1. Perwaiz MK. Interventional pulmonologist and thoracic surgeon: a difficult but necessary relationship. J Bronchology Interv Pulmonol 2017;24(1):e1.
2. Chen-Yoshikawa TF, Fukui T, Nakamura S, et al. J Med Sci 2020;82:161–74.

# Novel Screening Tools for Lung Cancer

Ju Ae Park, MD[a], Kei Suzuki, MD, MS[b,*]

**KEYWORDS**

• Lung cancer screening • Novel screening • Plasma biomarker • Airway biomarker • Breath printing

**KEY POINTS**

- Biomarkers found in plasma, sputum, and airway samples show promise as possible adjunctive studies to lung cancer screening.
- Plasma markers such as cell free DNA methylation in Lung EpiCheck and tumor-associated autoantibodies in EarlyCDT-Lung assays have demonstrated the predictive ability to detect lung cancer with limited sensitivity and specificities.
- Studies of bronchial and nasal epithelium have demonstrated the presence of tumor markers and positive findings for further development of lung cancer risk stratifying tools.
- Future studies of biomarkers in sputum such as methylation changes, microRNA, and tumor-associated autoantibodies have the potential to develop into more definitive adjunctive screening studies for lung cancer.

## INTRODUCTION

Lung cancer is the leading cause of cancer deaths, with an estimated 1.8 million deaths worldwide in 2020.[1] The overall 5-year survival rate for stage I non-small cell lung cancer (NSCLC) treated surgically is approximately 83%. However, in stark contrast, the 5-year survival rate for stage III and IV NSCLC remains at only 37% and 5.4%, respectively,[2] highlighting the critical importance of lung cancer screening to detect these diseases at an earlier stage. The current standard of care for lung cancer screening in the United States remains low-dose computed tomography (LDCT). The National Lung Screening Trial (NLST) reported that the annual LDCT screening leads to an overall 20% reduction in lung cancer-specific mortality compared to screening performed by chest X-ray. Despite the significant relative reduction in lung cancer mortality, the NLST results also showed a low cancer detection rate (1.1%).

Furthermore, even with the recently updated eligibility criteria, ~35% of patients harboring lung cancer would not meet the criteria to be screened.[3] This highlights the need to improve upon the current screening strategy. A good screening test is ideally easy to administer with minimal discomfort while having high reliability and validity. Several potential screening tools have been investigated, spanning from the airway, sputum/breath, to blood (**Fig. 1**). These tests aim to detect byproducts of lung cancer or provide risk-stratification tools that assess one's risk of harboring lung cancer. We herein review novel tools that have the potential of becoming adjuncts to current lung cancer screening.

## BIOMARKERS IN PLASMA FOR RISK STRATIFICATION OF LUNG CANCER

Several blood-based biomarkers are in the process of development or trials to determine their significance in lung cancer screening. The 3 most relevant at this time are plasma miRNA (microRNA), cell-free DNA methylation, and autoantibodies (**Table 1**).

[a] Department of General Surgery, Inova Fairfax Medical Campus, 3300 Gallows Road, Falls Church, VA 22042, USA; [b] Inova Thoracic Surgery, Schar Cancer Institute, 8081 Innovation Park Drive, Fairfax, VA 22031, USA
* Corresponding author.
*E-mail address:* Kei.suzuki@inova.org

Thorac Surg Clin 33 (2023) 215–226
https://doi.org/10.1016/j.thorsurg.2023.04.011

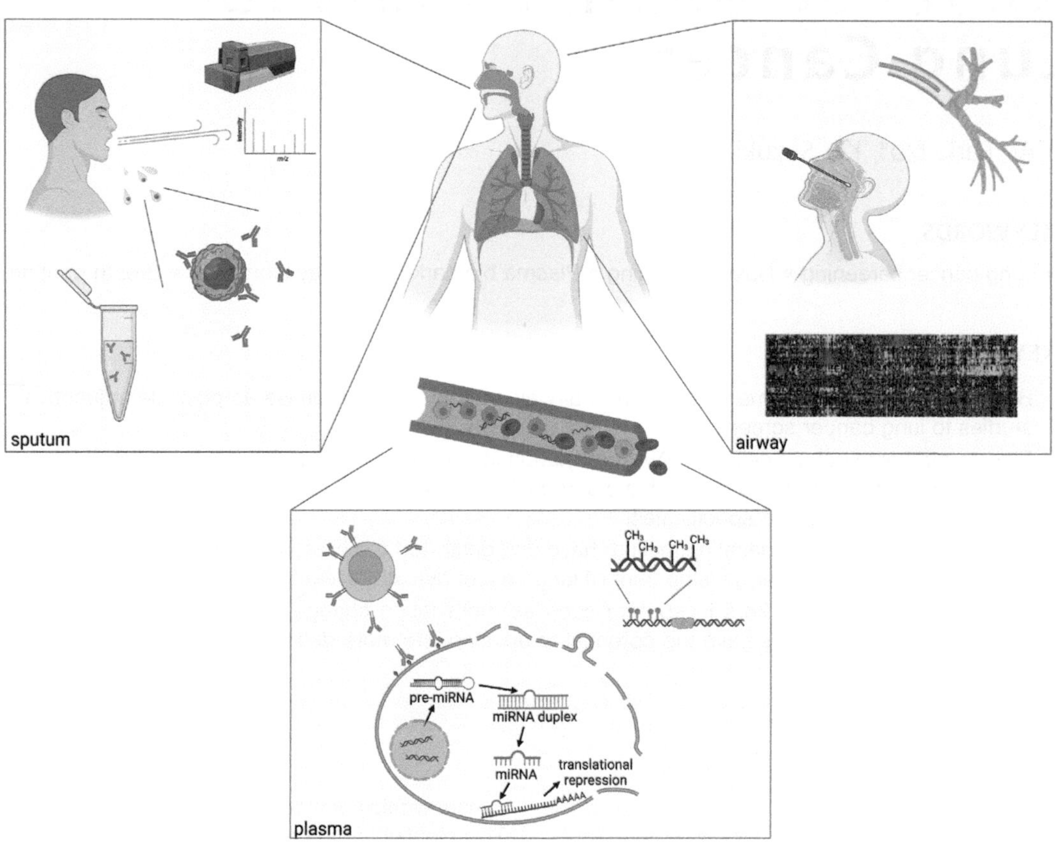


**Fig. 1.** Novel lung cancer screening technologies. Sputum: tumor associated autoantibodies obtained from sputum samples. Plasma: cell related micro-RNA, tumor associated autoantibodies, and DNA methylation changes. Airway: bronchial and nasal epithelium, volatile organic compound study via mass spectrometry.

## *MicroRNA*

Throughout the years, studies of routine biomarkers for lung cancer have resulted in various factors with differing sensitivities and specificities of correlation. More recently, miRNAs, also known as nonprotein coding RNAs, have come to light as potential biomarkers. miRNAs function as gene expression regulators and promote gene silencing by binding to mRNAs, subsequently causing translational repression or destabilization.[4] These molecules sustain active roles in regulating proliferative signaling, angiogenesis, apoptosis, genomic stability, and the inflammatory cascade. Dysfunction of any of these paths can lead to the induction of oncogenic behaviors and has been found to have significance in the pathogenesis of lung cancer.[5]

Upregulation of onco-miRNAs has been associated with chemo-resistance and increased risk of lung cancer.[6] Certain onco-miRNAs can also be utilized as diagnostic tools for certain types of cancers, as exemplified by Lebanony and colleagues,[7] who identified one miRNA (hsa-miR-205) highly specific for squamous cell carcinoma of the lung by collecting anonymized NSCLC tumor samples and performing miRNA profiling of 122 samples. These findings allowed for the establishment of a diagnostic protocol further validated by an independent set of 95 NSCLC tumor samples collected from 2 different institutions and was found to have a sensitivity and specificity of 96% and 79%, respectively, for identifying squamous cell carcinoma. Downregulation of tumor suppressive miRNAs has also been found to have significance in lung cancer. Yuan and colleagues[8] found reduced levels of miR-153 in cell lines and human tissue samples to be associated with increased expression of AKT, which promotes tumor growth in lung cancer tissues compared to adjacent control tissues. The downregulation of another miRNA (miR-218) known to have effects on cell migration and invasion ability was also related to advanced clinical staging and metastases in NSCLC by Shi and colleagues.[9] Analysis of 60 pairs of human NSCLC tissue samples and noncancerous lung tissue revealed significantly decreased levels of miRNA in cancerous tissue compared to noncancerous lung tissue as well as an inverse relationship of

**Table 1**
**Plasma biomarkers in lung cancer**

| Author | Study | Population | Method | Findings | Conclusion |
|---|---|---|---|---|---|
| Wang et al,[10] 2019 | miRNA | LC patients<br>*Control*—healthy or subjects with benign lung disease | Systematic review of 29 articles, 98 studies | *Pooled miRNA*: sens = 0.77, spec = 0.83 AUC = 0.87<br>*≥4 miRNA*: sens = 0.90, spec = 0.93, AUC = 0.97 | Panel of ≥4 miRNA combination results in high sensitivity/specificity for LC |
| Vykoukal et al,[11] 2022 | miRNA | LC patients—diagnosis within 1 y of blood draw<br>*Control*—matched controls with smoking history | Case control study from CARET trial data (high-risk population)<br>Case/control: n = 102/212 | *Three panel miRNA*: AUC = 0.63,sens = 22.6%, spec = 95%<br>*Four protein biomarker panel (4MP)*: AUC = 0.80, sens = 19%, spec = 95%<br>*combined miRNA +4MP*: AUC = 0.81, sens = 38.1%, spec = 95% | 3 miRNA panel + 4MP panel results in statistically significant increase in sensitivity of LC detection Δ19.1% (*P* = .006) |
| Ooki et al,[16] 2017 | DNA methylation | LC patients<br>*Control*—population matched subjects | Adenocarcinoma: n = 43<br>Squamous cell carcinoma: n = 40<br>Controls: n = 42 | *Stage IA adenocarcinoma*: sens = 72.1%, spec = 71.4%<br>*Stage IA squamous cell carcinoma*: sens = 60%, spec = 71.4% | Six gene methylation panel demonstrated comparable sensitivity and superior specificity to CT screening in detection of stage IA adenocarcinoma |
| Gaga et al,[18] 2021 | DNA methylation | *Europe*: suspected/confirmed LC patients<br>*Controls*—present/former smokers ≥50 years old<br>*China*: suspected/confirmed LC<br>*Controls*—healthy volunteers | Europe case/control: n = 279/137<br>China case/control: n = 30/15 | Europe: AUC = 0.882, sens = 87.2%, spec = 64.2%<br>China: AUC = 0.899, sens = 76.7%, spec = 93.3% | Lung EpiCheck has favorable sensitivity/ specificities for detection of early-stage LC (stage I, II, IIIA) and demonstrates a statistically significant difference in detecting LC when compared to LC risk factors alone in high-risk patients |
| Chapman et al,[21] 2008 | TAAb | LC patients with nonmatched healthy controls | Case/control: n = 104/50 | Combination 7 TAAb assay sens = 76%, spec = 92% | Combination panel of 7 TAAbs results in higher sensitivity and specificity for LC |
| Boyle et al,[22] 2011 | TAAb | LC patients and matched controls | Case/control: n = 269 | AUC = 0.64<br>sens/spec = 37%/90%<br>No significant diff between LC stages | Reproducible results of 6 panel TAAb assay with higher specificity than low-dose CT |
| Jett et al,[23] 2014 | TAAb | Subjects at high risk of LC (age and smoking history) | n = 1613 | 25/61 patients with positive test<br>57% (8/14) NSCLC with positive test in stage I/II | Clinical practice results correlate with previous case control studies and can detect early-stage LC |

*Abbreviations:* AUC, area under the curve; LC, lung cancer; NSCLC, non-small cell lung cancer; Sens, sensitivity; Spec, specificity; TAAb, tumor-associated autoantibody.

miR-218 expression with histologic grade. Further *in vivo* analysis in mice correlated with the *in vitro* data by demonstrating larger tumors with inhibition of miR-218 than those in control mice. Interestingly, miRNA dysregulation has also been noted in tobacco smoking and asbestos exposure, both lung cancer risk factors.[6]

These tissue-based findings have resulted in studies looking into the feasibility of detecting and utilizing miRNA in plasma as a diagnostic tool for lung cancer. A literature review of 98 studies by Wang and colleagues[10] used subgroup analysis and meta-regression to analyze miRNA in both respiratory and plasma samples. They found the sensitivity and specificity of plasma-based miRNA were higher at 0.80 and 0.84, respectively, compared to respiratory miRNA at 0.72 and 0.82, respectively. Further analysis of the data led to the conclusion that a panel of 4 or more miRNA combinations resulted in high sensitivity and specificity of 0.90 and 0.93, respectively, for lung cancer and could potentially be utilized as an early diagnostic tool. More recently, an analysis of 30 miRNA selected from literature reviews for the predictive ability to identify lung cancer was collected from serum samples of 102 individuals with lung cancer and compared to a control population (matched per age, sex, and smoking history). These serum samples were collected up to 1 year prior to the lung cancer diagnosis by selecting from the CARET trial, which was a previous randomized control trial conducted to assess the safety and cancer prevention efficacy of ß-carotene and retinyl palmitate supplementation in high-risk patients (ever heavy smokers and smokers with significant asbestos exposures). An assay of 30 miRNAs was performed and narrowed down to 5 miRNAs with statistically significant elevated serum levels in lung cancer cases compared to matched controls. Ultimately, a 3 miRNA marker panel of miRNA molecules identified across multiple independent studies as having variable expression in lung cancer was differentiated for increased sensitivity in identifying lung cancer. The 3 molecules—miR-21-5p, miR-320a-3p, and miR-210-3p—were noted to have a statistically significant elevation in serum levels and resulted in the highest area under the curve (AUC) of 0.63 among various combined panels. When combined with a 4 protein marker panel consisting of CA125, CEA, CYFRA 21 to 1, and Pro-SFTPB (precursor form of surfactant protein B) and controlling for a high specificity of 95%, a statistically significant improvement in sensitivity from 19% to 38.1% ($P$ = .006) was demonstrated compared to the sensitivity of detection with solely the 4 protein marker panel.[11] This predictive performance, when applied to a screening test, would allow for improved identification of lung cancer with a decreased risk of false positive results. There still exists a need to further evaluate and validate these studies in various populations and clinical scenarios; however, these studies provide a positive trajectory in elucidating improved tools for detecting lung cancer.

## Cell-Free DNA Methylation

Another available blood biomarker of interest is DNA methylation. DNA methylation plays various roles in genomics ranging from germline inactivation and tissue-specific gene expression to maintaining chromosome stability. In particular, methylation plays a role in cancer genomics by aberrant methylation of tumor suppressor genes leading to transcriptional silencing of said gene.[12] Hypermethylation of the promoter regions of tumor suppressor genes is noted to be a major contributor to epimutation driving oncogenesis.[13] Examples of this have been found in retinoblastoma, colorectal, and renal cancers.[14]

Cell-free DNA with methylation changes can be detected in cancer patients' serum and other body fluids.[12] These fragments of free DNA circulating in plasma range in size from 80 to 200 base pairs and are also found to be elevated in other diseases such as lupus. They are thought to be both spontaneously secreted by tumors or passively generated by the destruction of tumor cells.[15] Various methylation biomarkers have been found to be correlated with lung cancer, and these combined can be formed into a panel of methylation regions that could increase the sensitivity and specificity of these studies. For example, Ooki and colleagues[16] determined a 6 gene methylation panel for lung cancer detection and risk stratification. An epigenome-wide analysis of lung adenocarcinoma samples selected from The Cancer Genome Atlas dataset (TCGA) was first analyzed, and 30 genes with differentially methylated regions associated with lung cancer were selected. Evaluation of these 30 genes led to a selection of 6 genes with higher methylation rates in tumor samples and ranged in sensitivity from 62.5% to 87.5% in a setting of 100% specificity. Given these findings, serum samples from stage IA adenocarcinoma (n = 43), stage IA squamous cell carcinoma (n = 40), and population-matched controls (n = 42) were obtained, and assessment of the methylation gene panel revealed a sensitivity and specificity of 72.1% and 71.4%, respectively, for stage IA adenocarcinoma along with a sensitivity of 60% for stage IA squamous cell carcinoma.

More recently, a methylation panel utilized in urine-based bladder EpiCheck was able to demonstrate a 92% sensitivity and 88% specificity for high-grade urothelial carcinoma in the surveillance of bladder cancer patients.[17] Based on this concept, a lung cancer-specific panel of 6 methylation biomarkers was developed from a possible 485,000 different candidate markers and tested at various sites across Europe and a single site in China.[18] A case–control study was utilized by collecting blood specimens from subjects with pathologically proven primary lung cancer or suspected lung cancer undergoing a diagnostic procedure. These cases (n = 179) were compared with 2 different sets of control populations in China and Europe with the exclusion criteria of present or prior history of cancer. PCR amplified samples were analyzed and given EpiScores reflecting the methylation level in the assay markers. The overall sensitivity/specificity of the panel was 87.2% (81.3%–91.7%)/64.2% (55.6%–72.2%) with AUC 0.882 (0.846–0.918). Maximizing for sensitivity with low cut-off, Lung EpiCheck detected NSCLC stages I, II, and IIIA with 85.1% (76.7%–91.4%) sensitivity, whereas it was able to detect stage I NSCLC with 78.4% (61.8%–90.2%) sensitivity. The predictive ability of EpiScore was evaluated against lung cancer risk factors alone (age, sex, smoking status, pack-years, chronic obstructive pulmonary disease [COPD]) versus risk factors in combination with EpiScore among a subset of patients with full smoking history. This demonstrated a significantly increased AUC of 0.942 (0.13–0.971) from an AUC of 0.852 (0.805–0.900) with a *P*-value of less than 0.0001. This all demonstrates the strong performance of Lung EpiCheck in the predictive ability for lung cancer.[18]

Because of certain limitations encountered as a consequence of data collection limitations, there is a need for further validation studies for this panel. However, it is a promising study that could make way for an adjunctive screening test to the current standards with LDCT in patients with a high risk of lung cancer.

### Autoantibodies

Although cancer cells are known to avoid immune recognition, innate expression of proteins, also known as tumor-associated antigens (TAA), and their release from tumor cells naturally trigger an immune response to varying degrees. The advent of technologies in proteomic methods has allowed for the detection of new antibody biomarkers to be studied in relation to cancer.[19] Well-known TAA TP53 has been extensively studied and was shown to induce the formation of tumor-associated autoantibodies (TAAbs), which are highly correlated with the presence of various types of cancer even while controlling for age, gender, smoking, and cumulative asbestos exposure in serum samples of patients exposed to asbestos. One hundred fifteen patients with relatively high cumulative asbestos exposure were followed for incidence of subsequent cancer development for 22 to 23 years, and serum samples obtained from those within the cohort who developed cancer were studied for the presence of TAAbs to TP53. Univariate analysis demonstrated a statistically significant ($P$ = .0015) association between p53 autoantibodies and cancer in the patients with asbestos exposures who developed cancer, the majority of which was lung cancer.[20] Other studies have identified the presence of autoantibodies in the serum of lung cancer patients up to 5 years before screening CT scans were obtained.[19] This has led to the evaluation of a 7 panel TAA assay for autoantibodies in lung cancer by obtaining plasma samples at various time points after diagnosis from 104 patients with confirmed cancer and 50 healthy donors as controls (nonmatched). The combination panel was determined to have a sensitivity of 76% and specificity of 92% for lung cancer for all samples. In the subset of data in patients within 1 and 6 months of diagnosis and prior to treatment, the sensitivities of the panel for detection of lung cancer remained at 68% and 74%, respectively.[21] The validity of this screening process was confirmed when Boyle and colleagues[22] obtained serum samples of newly diagnosed lung cancer patients and healthy controls with no prior malignant disease (matched by gender, age, and smoking history) in 3 different groups, which were then assessed for the presence of TAAbs. The autoantibody assay was verified to identify 40% of primary lung cancers with a specificity of 90% against the control population. This assay was formatted into a trademarked assay, EarlyCDT-Lung, which was ultimately studied in routine clinical practice (n = 1699) and detected all-stage lung cancers with a sensitivity of 41% and specificity of 87%, which is congruent to prior studies and analyses.[23] The study carries a high specificity, allowing for improved differentiation between benign and malignant nodules. However, because of the low sensitivity, this assay would not be a recommended isolated screening test for lung cancer. With so many validating studies, EarlyCDT-Lung and similar assays seem promising to become the next adjunctive study for the early determination of lung cancer in high-risk individuals.

## MOLECULAR CHANGES IN THE AIRWAY AS POTENTIAL RISK-STRATIFICATION TOOL FOR LUNG CANCER

Lung carcinogenesis is thought to be in part due to injury imparted by inhalants such as cigarette smoke. Based on the "field of injury" hypothesis that proposes that an inhalant causes a molecular response throughout the respiratory tract, epithelial cells in the airway present a potential screening tool for lung cancer. Using high-throughput technologies to study the molecular changes imparted by such exposure has resulted in potentially promising tools for diagnosing lung cancer (**Table 2**).

In the AEGIS study, Silvestri and colleagues[24] evaluated the molecular changes in the bronchial epithelium in patients with suspicious lung nodules undergoing bronchoscopy.[25] In this multicenter trial, 639 patients undergoing bronchoscopy for suspected lung cancer were enrolled. Of this, 272 (43%) bronchoscopies were nondiagnostic, of which 120 patients were ultimately diagnosed with lung cancer. With the addition of the gene expression classifier developed from the bronchial epithelium obtained by brushing, the sensitivity was 96% to 98%, compared with 74% to 76% for bronchoscopy alone ($P < .001$). Furthermore, in patients deemed by clinicians to be at intermediate risk for lung cancer (10%–60%), bronchoscopy alone was nondiagnostic in 83% despite 41% eventually being diagnosed with lung cancer. In this group, the airway classifier had a negative predictive value of 91%.

Building on this finding, the AEGIS team investigated whether a nasal rather than bronchial epithelium would provide similar results, given that they both represent the airway epithelium.[26] In a cohort of 375 current and former smokers with suspicious imaging findings, nasal epithelium brushings were prospectively collected. In total, 535 genes were identified to be differentially expressed in the nasal epithelium of patients diagnosed with lung cancer compared to those with benign disease. Genes downregulated in patients with lung cancer were enriched for genes associated with DNA damage, apoptosis regulation, and processes involved in immune system activation, including the interferon-gamma signaling pathway and antigen presentation. In contrast, genes upregulated in patients with lung cancer were enriched for endocytosis and iron transport genes. The genes with cancer-associated expression in nasal epithelium were split into upregulated and downregulated gene sets. They were subsequently examined for their distribution within all genes ranked from most downregulated to most upregulated in the bronchial epithelium of patients with cancer using gene set enrichment analysis. The genes with increased expression in nasal epithelium were enriched among the genes most induced in the bronchial epithelium of patients with cancer ($P < .001$). At the same time, the reverse was true for genes with decreased expression in nasal epithelium ($P < .001$). This suggests the presence of a highly concordant lung cancer field of injury that is shared in both bronchial and nasal tissues. Collectively, these data support the "field of injury" theory that cancer-associated gene expression differences can be seen in the normal airway epithelium, including both the bronchus and nasal epithelium.

Similar to the bronchial biomarker, using a training set of 375 samples from the AEGIS cohort, a 37 gene clinical-molecular biomarker was developed that uses the Gould clinical risk model as a starting point and incorporates genes whose expression in nasal epithelium is associated with lung cancer, together with other genes whose expression is associated with clinical risk factors in the Gould model (such as smoking status and years of smoking cessation in former smokers) as well as actual clinical factors for which we could not derive gene expression correlates (such as age and mass size). The performance of this clinical-molecular model was validated in an independent set of 130 nasal samples. The clinical-molecular model yielded an AUC of 0.81 in the validation set, significantly higher than the AUC of 0.74 achieved by the clinical model alone ($P = .05$). More importantly, adding cancer-associated gene expression to the clinical risk factor model resulted in a significant increase in sensitivity from 0.79 to 0.91 and an increase in negative predictive value from 0.73 to 0.85. This demonstrates that nasal gene expression captures molecular information about the likelihood of lung cancer independent of clinical factors and therefore has the potential to improve upon clinical models for lung cancer detection.

The field of injury hypothesis has shown promising results in risk stratifying for lung cancer in the setting of suspicious lung nodules. Similar approaches in patients yet to receive screening CT may provide a potential risk-stratification tool that can be used as an adjunct to lung cancer screening. In addition, the nasal epithelium would allow for ease of collection.

## *Breath Prints*

Breath analysis of volatile organic compounds (VOC) for lung cancer screening is a rapidly developing field. Detection and characterization of VOC can be approached in 2 ways. Individual VOC can be identified as associated with lung cancer (or any disease process of interest), usually by gas chromatography-mass spectrometry.[27] This method transfers a gas sample into gas chromatography-mass spectrometry. It is analyzed according to the chromatography column's time to elution (ie, absorption) and the

**Table 2**
**Breath and sputum biomarkers in lung cancer**

| Author | Study | Population | Method | Findings | Conclusion |
|---|---|---|---|---|---|
| Silvestri et al,[24] 2015 | Bronchial epithelium gene expression | Current/former smokers undergoing bronchoscopy for evaluation of suspicious pulmonary lesions | Two multicenter prospective studies<br>AEGIS-1: n = 298<br>AEGIS-2: n = 341 | AEGIS-1: AUC = 0.78, sens = 88%, spec = 47%<br>AEGIS-2: AUC = 0.74, sens = 89%, spec = 47%<br>Combination classifier + bronchoscopy<br>AEGIS-1: sens = 96%<br>AEGIS-2: sens = 98% | Gene-expression classifier as adjunct to bronchoscopy improves diagnostic performance |
| AEGIS Study Team[26] 2017 | Nasal epithelium gene expression | Current/former smokers undergoing bronchoscopy for evaluation of suspicious pulmonary lesions | Nasal: n = 554<br>Bronchial: n = 299<br>Validation set: n = 130 | Statistically significant ($P < .001$) concordant gene expression alterations between nasal and bronchial epithelium<br>Validation set: AUC = 0.81, sens = 91%, spec = 52% | There exists a correlation between cancer-associated genes in nasal and bronchial epithelium.<br>The addition of LC-associated gene expression to clinical risk factors increases sensitivity in LC detection |
| McWilliams et al,[32] 2015 | Volatile organic compounds in exhaled breath | LC patients.<br>*Control*—high risk smokers | Case/control: n = 25/166 | 80% accuracy of e-nose in distinguishing LC patients from high-risk controls | VOCs may have clinical utility in LC screening |
| Rocco et al,[33] 2016 | Volatile organic compounds in exhaled breath | High-risk patients—55–75 y current/former smokers, known carcinogen exposure, COPD | Validation study of BIONOTE<br>n = 100 | AUC = 0.87 ($P = .0008$)<br>Sens = 86%<br>Spec = 95% | Because of high specificity, VOC may be utilized as an adjunctive test to LDCT to reduce false positive rates |
| Gasparri et al,[34] 2016 | Volatile organic compounds in exhaled breath | Confirmed LC patients and healthy matched controls | Case/control: n = 70/76 | Sens = 81%<br>Spec = 91%<br>Largest sens = 92% with stage I | VOCs can differentiate LC patients from healthy controls |

(*continued on next page*)

**Table 2**
**(*continued*)**

| Author | Study | Population | Method | Findings | Conclusion |
|---|---|---|---|---|---|
| Shlomi et al,[35] 2017 | Volatile organic compounds in exhaled breath | LC patients<br>*Control*—patients with benign nodules | Case/control: n = 89/30 | 87% accuracy in discriminating LC from benign nodules, PPV = 87.7%, NPV = 87.5%<br>EGFR mutation discrimination: accuracy = 83%, sens = 79%, spec = 85% | VOCs can detect LC from benign masses and EGFR mutations from wild type |
| Su et al,[50] 2016 | Sputum small nucleolar RNA | LC patients<br>*Control*—cancer-free smokers | Case/control:<br>Training set: n = 59/61<br>Validation set: n = 67/69 | Training: sens = 74.8%, spec = 83.6%<br>Validation: sens = 74.63%, spec = 84.06% | Small nucleolar RNAs are detectable in sputum and have the ability to differentiate for LC |
| Li et al,[51] 2021 | Sputum TAAb | LC patients<br>Control—cancer-free smokers | Case/control:<br>Discovery set: n = 30/30<br>Validation set: n = 166/213 | Combined 3 TAAb biomarker panel:<br>AUC = 0.88<br>Sens = 81%, spec = 83% | TAAb panel in sputum have potential as biomarkers for LC |

*Abbreviations:* AUC, area under the curve; LC, lung cancer; LDCT, low-dose computed tomography; NPV, negative predictive value; PPV, positive predictive value; Sens, sensitivity; Spec, specificity; TAAb, tumor-associated autoantibody; VOC, volatile organic compounds.

mass-to-charge ratio. The main downside of this approach is that no VOC uniquely associated with lung cancer exists. Also, quantifying VOCs by gas chromatography-mass spectrometry is an expensive, time-consuming process that demands expert personnel and dedicated laboratory facilities. In addition, lung cancer biomarkers identified by this approach are largely inconsistent. For example, in one study, 22 VOCs were associated with lung cancer,[28] whereas in another study, 16 VOCs were associated with lung cancer.[29] Other authors have concluded that VOC analysis by gas chromatography-mass spectrometry cannot reliably distinguish between those with or without lung cancer.[30,31]

Alternatively, one can look for exhaled breath fingerprints through cross-reactive sensors to define specific patterns of disease-related VOCs. The technology can differ by the sensing material and the array composition. The so-called e-nose, as it reproduces the combinatorial selectivity of the human nose, can be used to derive a "breath print," similar to a fingerprint that is unique to each individual. This can then be assessed for their associations with a disease state of interest, such as lung cancer. The e-nose has been tested clinically with the goal of early lung cancer detection. McWilliams and colleagues[32] investigated the utility of e-nose in 25 patients with lung cancer and 166 high-risk smokers without lung cancer. In their study, e-nose could distinguish patients with lung cancer from high-risk controls with a better than 80% classification accuracy. Rocco and colleagues[33] validated their platform BIONOTE in 100 high-risk individuals, yielding a sensitivity of 86% and specificity of 95%. Gasparri and colleagues[34] studied 70 patients with lung cancer along with 76 healthy controls and demonstrated 81% sensitivity and 91% specificity. In another study, Shlomi and colleagues[35] utilized e-nose in 119 patients, of which 30 had benign nodules and 89 had lung cancer. Discrimination of early lung cancer from benign nodules had 87% accuracy and positive and negative predictive values of 87.7% and 87.5%, respectively. Furthermore, they could distinguish lung cancer patients with epidermal growth factor receptor (EGFR) mutation (n = 19) from those with wild-type EGFR (n = 34) with an accuracy of 83%, sensitivity of 79%, and specificity of 85%. These studies show the promise of e-nose in distinguishing benign from malignant lung nodules and its potential utility as an adjunctive tool for lung cancer screening in a high-risk population.

Although early data are promising, the existing technology uses complex, expensive, and low-throughput analytical platforms, preventing its applicability for mass screening. The reliability of a new portable device to enable rapid onsite lung cancer diagnosis will be necessary.

## BIOMARKERS IN SPUTUM FOR RISK STRATIFICATION OF LUNG CANCER

Sputum testing for cancer detection is theoretically a favorable method that can be a noninvasive and nonradiological technique for lung cancer screening. Research has shown an established association between abnormal sputum production and lung cancer.[36] Previous research has also demonstrated sputum testing to be cost-effective and likely to be covered by third-party payors.[37,38] Sputum can be easily collected by patients at home or any clinical setting and induced or collected spontaneously. Ideally, the samples contain alveolar macrophages or bronchial epithelial cells, which confirm the samples originate deep within the lung.[39]

Sputum cytology testing involves identifying aberrant cell morphology in the sample and was first utilized for lung cancer diagnostics in the 1960s.[36,40] However, early studies failed to show an advantage in lung cancer detection or survival. A randomized study of the addition of sputum cytology/cytometry testing to LDCT conducted from 2007 to 2011 failed to improve the efficiency of lung cancer screening.[41] A 2003 review article of 16 studies on sputum cytology, including more than 28,000 patients, reported a range of 42% to 97% sensitivity, with an average sensitivity of 66%, and an average specificity of 99%.[42] Modern cytology methods, such as computer-assisted image analysis, have increased sensitivity up to 97% and significantly reduced false positive and false negative rates.[43] In many developed countries, tumor biopsies have replaced the use of sputum cytology for making a lung cancer diagnosis. In lesser-developed regions, sputum cytology is an affordable diagnostic tool and is still implemented in clinical practice.[44,45]

Apart from cytology, other biomarker methods are available for detecting and evaluating lung cancer in a sputum sample using molecular analysis techniques (see **Table 2**). The possible applications for a biomarker sputum test include (i) the identification of at-risk individuals who should be screened using LDCT; (ii) after an LDCT scan reveals a solid lesion, a sputum biomarker for use as a diagnostic test for malignancy; and (iii) after an LDCT scan shows a ground glass lesion, it can be assessed for the risk of becoming malignant. A risk marker can identify those at risk of developing malignancy without measurable disease present and may be a measure of exposure to carcinogens and the development of carcinoma *in situ*.[46] In patients with current symptomatic lung cancer, a sputum test may be useful for diagnostic workup of malignancy and to perform predictive analysis for treatment response or survival.[47] Detecting genetic aberrations in sputum, including methylation in commonly suppressed genes in lung cancer, can also be a method of early detection in those at high risk for lung cancer, particularly smokers or those with COPD.[48] Additional research has shown that microRNAs and dysregulation of small nucleolar RNAs play a vital role in lung tumor development.[49] In an analysis of small nucleolar RNAs in sputum by qRT-PCR, this biomarker had a significantly higher sensitivity (74.58%) compared with sputum cytology (45.76%) for detecting lung cancer.[50] More recently, a study by Li and colleagues[51] demonstrated the potential of TAAbs in detecting NSCLC. This is based on the prior plasma studies of TAAbs with the speculation that a direct sample from the respiratory tract could increase the test's sensitivity as this is theoretically close to the tumor source. Initially, 8 out of 28 lung antigens were identified and validated to have augmented or reduced interaction levels with TAAbs in patients with lung cancer versus cancer-free smokers. From this, an optimal panel of 3 TAAbs was selected, and subsequent analysis of these 3 markers demonstrated an AUC of 0.88 in distinguishing NSCLC and a sensitivity and specificity of 81% and 83%, respectively. Although this was a small study with limited sensitivity, it shows positive findings that could lead to further investigations. Currently, no singular, approved sputum-based biomarker is utilized in lung cancer screening, and research efforts continue to be underway.

Although the previously discussed sputum cytology has habitually failed to yield adequate and representative samples for reliable lung cancer screening, the arrival of modern image analysis algorithms, in combination with artificial intelligence, may be a promising diagnostic tool in the future.[52] Three-dimensional cell imaging technology, using sputum samples enriched for bronchial epithelial cells, can identify abnormal cells in sputum samples of screened patients.[53] This test may be used as a primary screening modality with a reported sensitivity of 90% when at least 800 bronchial cells are collected for analysis or are used concomitantly with LDCT.[54] When this testing is used to supplement LDCT, fewer cells are typically required as the clinician can assimilate clinical and molecular data with imaging results for greater diagnostic accuracy.[52] Modern advances in genetic and nuclear image analyses show great potential in the refinement of diagnosis beyond that attained with conventional sputum cytology examination.

## SUMMARY

Although LDCTs have been shown to decrease lung cancer mortality, one area of improvement is better identification of the high-risk population, which could lead to improved cancer detection by imaging. Several tests at different stages of development can serve as adjuncts to imaging in the screening process for lung cancer. Tests developed from blood, airway, breath, and sputum samples represent easy-to-collect, nonradiation tools and hold promise as potential adjuncts to screening. Continued studies, including a synergistic approach using molecular biomarkers, imaging, and artificial intelligence technology in developing less costly and easily accessible screening studies, would benefit the goal of early detection and intervention and ultimately improve patient outcomes.

## DISCLOSURE

The authors do not have any commercial or financial conflicts of interest to disclose.

## ACKNOWLEDGMENTS

The authors would like to thank Wayne Pereanu for his assistance in formulating this article.

## REFERENCES

1. Ferlay J, E. M., Lam F, Colombet M, Mery L, Piñeros M, et al. Lung Fact Sheet, Available at: https://gco.iarc.fr/today/data/factsheets/cancers/15-Lung-fact-sheet.pdf. 2020. Accessed November 17, 2022.
2. NCI. SEER Cancer Stat Facts: Lung and Bronchus Cancer, Available at: https://seer.cancer.gov/statfacts/html/lungb.html. Accessed November 17, 2022.
3. Pu CY, Lusk CM, Neslund-Dudas C, et al. Comparison Between the 2021 USPSTF Lung Cancer Screening Criteria and Other Lung Cancer Screening Criteria for Racial Disparity in Eligibility, *JAMA Oncol*, 8, 2022, 374–382.
4. Bartel DP. MicroRNAs: target recognition and regulatory functions. Cell 2009;136:215–33.
5. Wu KL, Tsai YM, Lien CT, et al. The Roles of MicroRNA in Lung Cancer. Int J Mol Sci 2019;20. https://doi.org/10.3390/ijms20071611.
6. Sheervalilou R, Shahraki O, Hasanifard L, et al. Electrochemical Nano-biosensors as Novel Approach for the Detection of Lung Cancer-related MicroRNAs, *Curr Mol Med*, 20, 2019, 13–35.

7. Lebanony D, Benjamin H, Gilad S, et al. Diagnostic assay based on hsa-miR-205 expression distinguishes squamous from nonsquamous non-small-cell lung carcinoma. J Clin Oncol 2009;27:2030–7.
8. Yuan Y, Du W, Wang Y, et al. Suppression of AKT expression by miR-153 produced anti-tumor activity in lung cancer. Int J Cancer 2015;136:1333–40.
9. Shi ZM, Wang L, Shen H, et al. Downregulation of miR-218 contributes to epithelial-mesenchymal transition and tumor metastasis in lung cancer by targeting Slug/ZEB2 signaling. Oncogene 2017;36: 2577–88.
10. Wang Y, Guan J, Wang Y. Could microRNA be used as a diagnostic tool for lung cancer? J Cell Biochem 2019;120:18937–45.
11. Vykoukal J, Fahrmann JF, Patel N, et al. Contributions of Circulating microRNAs for Early Detection of Lung Cancer. Cancers 2022;14. https://doi.org/10.3390/cancers14174221.
12. Kristensen LS, Hansen LL. PCR-based methods for detecting single-locus DNA methylation biomarkers in cancer diagnostics, prognostics, and response to treatment. Clin Chem 2009;55:1471–83.
13. Nishiyama A, Nakanishi M. Navigating the DNA methylation landscape of cancer. Trends Genet 2021;37:1012–27.
14. Herman JG, Baylin SB. Gene silencing in cancer in association with promoter hypermethylation. N Engl J Med 2003;349:2042–54.
15. Li L, Fu K, Zhou W, et al. Applying circulating tumor DNA methylation in the diagnosis of lung cancer. Precis Clin Med 2019;2:45–56.
16. Ooki A, Maleki Z, Tsay JC, et al. A Panel of Novel Detection and Prognostic Methylated DNA Markers in Primary Non-Small Cell Lung Cancer and Serum DNA. Clin Cancer Res 2017;23:7141–52.
17. Witjes JA, Morote J, Cornel E, et al. Performance of the Bladder EpiCheck Methylation Test for Patients Under Surveillance for Non-muscle-invasive Bladder Cancer: Results of a Multicenter, Prospective. Blinded Clinical Trial, Eur Urol Oncol 2018;1:307–13.
18. Gaga M, Chorostowska-Wynimko J, Horvath I, et al. Validation of Lung EpiCheck, a novel methylation-based blood assay, for the detection of lung cancer in European and Chinese high-risk individuals. Eur Respir J 2021;57:2021. https://doi.org/10.1183/13993003.02682-2020.
19. Desmetz C, Mange A, Maudelonde T, et al. Autoantibody signatures: progress and perspectives for early cancer detection. J Cell Mol Med 2011;15: 2013–24.
20. Li Y, Karjalainen A, Koskinen H, et al. p53 autoantibodies predict subsequent development of cancer. Int J Cancer 2005;114:157–60.
21. Chapman CJ, Murray A, McElveen JE, et al. Autoantibodies in lung cancer: possibilities for early detection and subsequent cure. Thorax 2008;63:228–33.
22. Boyle P, Chapman CJ, Holdenrieder S, et al. Clinical validation of an autoantibody test for lung cancer. Ann Oncol 2011;22:383–9.
23. Jett JR, Peek LJ, Fredericks L, et al. Audit of the autoantibody test, EarlyCDT(R)-lung, in 1600 patients: an evaluation of its performance in routine clinical practice. Lung Cancer 2014;83:51–5.
24. Silvestri GA, Vachani A, Whitney D, et al. A Bronchial Genomic Classifier for the Diagnostic Evaluation of Lung Cancer. N Engl J Med 2015;373:243–51.
25. Spira A, Beane JE, Shah V, et al. Airway epithelial gene expression in the diagnostic evaluation of smokers with suspect lung cancer, *Nat Med*, 13, 2007, 361–366.
26. Team AS. Shared Gene Expression Alterations in Nasal and Bronchial Epithelium for Lung Cancer Detection. J Natl Cancer Inst 2017;109.
27. Rocco G, Pennazza G, Santonico M, et al. Breathprinting and Early Diagnosis of Lung Cancer, *J Thorac Oncol*, 13, 2018, 883–894.
28. Phillips M, Gleeson K, Hughes JM, et al. Volatile organic compounds in breath as markers of lung cancer: a cross-sectional study. Lancet 1999;353:1930–3.
29. Phillips M, Altorki N, Austin JH, et al. Prediction of lung cancer using volatile biomarkers in breath, *Cancer Biomark*, 3, 2007, 95–109.
30. Kischkel S, Miekisch W, Sawacki A, et al. Breath biomarkers for lung cancer detection and assessment of smoking related effects–confounding variables, influence of normalization and statistical algorithms. Clin Chim Acta 2010;411:1637–44.
31. Schallschmidt K, Becker R, Jung C, et al. Comparison of volatile organic compounds from lung cancer patients and healthy controls-challenges and limitations of an observational study. J Breath Res 2016; 10:046007.
32. McWilliams A, Beigi P, Srinidhi A, et al. Sex and Smoking Status Effects on the Early Detection of Early Lung Cancer in High-Risk Smokers Using an Electronic Nose. IEEE Trans Biomed Eng 2015;62: 2044–54.
33. Rocco R, Incalzi RA, Pennazza G, et al. BIONOTE e-nose technology may reduce false positives in lung cancer screening programmesdagger, *Eur J Cardio Thorac Surg*, 49, 2016, 1112–1117, [discussion: 1117].
34. Gasparri R, Santonico M, Valentini C, et al. Volatile signature for the early diagnosis of lung cancer. J Breath Res 2016;10:016007.
35. Shlomi D, Abud M, Liran O, et al. Detection of Lung Cancer and EGFR Mutation by Electronic Nose System. J Thorac Oncol 2017;12:1544–51.
36. Prindiville SA, Byers T, Hirsch FR, et al. Sputum cytological atypia as a predictor of incident lung cancer in a cohort of heavy smokers with airflow obstruction. Cancer Epidemiol Biomarkers Prev 2003;12: 987–93.

37. Raab SS, Hornberger J, Raffin T. The importance of sputum cytology in the diagnosis of lung cancer: a cost-effectiveness analysis. Chest 1997;112:937–45.
38. Ramaswamy A. Lung Cancer Screening: Review and 2021 Update. Curr Pulmonol Rep 2022;11: 15–28.
39. Thunnissen FB. Sputum examination for early detection of lung cancer. J Clin Pathol 2003;56:805–10.
40. Tockman MS, Gupta PK, Myers JD, et al. Sensitive and specific monoclonal antibody recognition of human lung cancer antigen on preserved sputum cells: a new approach to early lung cancer detection. J Clin Oncol 1988;6:1685–93.
41. Spiro SG, Shah PL, Rintoul RC, et al. Sequential screening for lung cancer in a high-risk group: randomised controlled trial: LungSEARCH: a randomised controlled trial of Surveillance using sputum and imaging for the EARly detection of lung Cancer in a High-risk group. Eur Respir J 2019;54. https://doi.org/10.1183/13993003.00581-2019.
42. Schreiber G, McCrory DC. Performance characteristics of different modalities for diagnosis of suspected lung cancer: summary of published evidence. Chest 2003;123:115S–28S.
43. El-Baz A, Beache GM, Gimel'farb G, et al. Computer-aided diagnosis systems for lung cancer: challenges and methodologies, *Int J Biomed Imaging*, 2013, 942353, doi:10.1155/2013/942353(2013).
44. Ammanagi AS, Dombale VD, Miskin AT, et al. Sputum cytology in suspected cases of carcinoma of lung (Sputum cytology a poor man's bronchoscopy!). Lung India 2012;29:19–23.
45. Rivera MP, Mehta AC, American College of Chest P. Initial diagnosis of lung cancer: ACCP evidence-based clinical practice guidelines (2nd edition). Chest 2007;132:131S–48S.
46. Selamat SA, Galler JS, Joshi AD, et al. DNA methylation changes in atypical adenomatous hyperplasia, adenocarcinoma in situ, and lung adenocarcinoma. PLoS One 2011;6:e21443.
47. Hubers AJ, Prinsen CF, Sozzi G, et al. Molecular sputum analysis for the diagnosis of lung cancer. Br J Cancer 2013;109:530–7.
48. Tessema M, Tassew D, Yingling CM, et al. Identification of novel epigenetic abnormalities as sputum biomarkers for lung cancer risk among smokers and COPD patients. Lung Cancer 2020;146:189–96.
49. Sheervalilou R, Ansarin K, Aval SF, et al. An update on sputum MicroRNAs in lung cancer diagnosis. Diagn Cytopathol 2016;44:442–9.
50. Su J, Liao J, Gao L, et al. Analysis of small nucleolar RNAs in sputum for lung cancer diagnosis. Oncotarget 2016;7:5131–42.
51. Li N, Holden VK, Deepak J, et al. Autoantibodies against tumor-associated antigens in sputum as biomarkers for lung cancer. Transl Oncol 2021;14: 100991.
52. Seijo LM, Peled N, Ajona D, et al. Biomarkers in Lung Cancer Screening: Achievements, Promises, and Challenges, *J Thorac Oncol*, 14, 2019, 343–357.
53. Meyer MG, Hayenga JW, Neumann T, et al. The Cell-CT 3-dimensional cell imaging technology platform enables the detection of lung cancer using the noninvasive LuCED sputum test. Cancer Cytopathol 2015;123:512–23.
54. Nelson A, Meyer M, Katdare R, et al. Early detection of lung cancer based on three-dimensional, morphometric analysis of cells from sputum. J Clin Oncol 2014;32:7547.

# Intraoperative Molecular Imaging of Lung Cancer

Check for updates

Lye-Yeng Wong, MD, Natalie S. Lui, MD, MAS*

**KEYWORDS**

• Intraoperative molecular imaging • Fluorescence • Indocyanine green • EC 17 • OTL38
• Thoracic surgery

**KEY POINTS**

- Intraoperative molecular imaging (IMI) is a growing field and a promising adjunct for tumor localization, margin and lymph node assessment, and discovery of nodules unidentified by traditional imaging techniques.
- Imaging agents are either nontargeted or targeted, and they fluoresce in either the visible light spectrum or the near-infrared spectrum. Studies are focused on developing targeted agents in the near-infrared spectrum to capitalize on enhancing tumor tissue specificity with low background noise.
- Pafolacianine, or OTL38, is a folate receptor-$\alpha$-targeted probe that has shown great success in a multi-institutional phase 2 trial. OTL38 demonstrated the ability to modify operations, identify additional cancers, and upstage tumors intraoperatively. The ELUCIDATE trial is a phase 3 randomized clinical trial recently completed that will result soon.
- Antibody-based imaging receptors are on the horizon, and preclinical studies support the ongoing investigations in lung cancer.

## INTRODUCTION

As more emphasis is placed on preventive health measures, the rates of early-stage lung cancers detected through screening programs have increased. This increasing incidence, coupled by the awareness of surgical morbidity and importance of preserving pulmonary function, has in turn led to the growing use of both sublobar resections and minimally invasive techniques to provide a surgical cure. Sublobar resections, such as segmentectomy and wedge resections, can be curative in appropriate early-stage disease.[1,2] Tumor localization and resection with adequate margins are key aspects of these operations. With approximately 40% of all thoracic surgery cases now performed using minimally invasive techniques, tactile feedback is limited, which necessitates conversion to open surgery in 5% to 25% of cases.[3–5] Similarly, even with years of surgical experience, the naked eye cannot sufficiently detect microscopic cancer cells, which necessitates the use of pathologic frozen sections. Nevertheless, with these time- and cost-intensive techniques, the incidence of positive margins after lung cancer resections is still cited to be as high as 20%.[6] Each close or positive surgical margin adds $6000 to $129,000 to patient treatment costs, and more importantly, increases rates of recurrence and doubles the mortality rate.[7–9] Intraoperative molecular imaging (IMI) is an exciting field that bridges this gap and addresses many of the current limitations in thoracic surgery.

Currently, well-resourced institutions have existing methods to enhance tumor localization. Three-dimensional modeling of radiology images is one such example, but this tool requires time, specialized software, and personnel. This holds true for other described techniques, like preoperative placement of wires, coils, fiducials, and tracers,

Department of Cardiothoracic Surgery, Stanford University School of Medicine, 300 Pasteur Drive, Falk Building, Stanford, CA 94305, USA
* Corresponding author.
*E-mail address:* natalielui@stanford.edu
Twitter: @LyeYengWongMD (L.-Y.W.); @natalielui22 (N.S.L.)

Thorac Surg Clin 33 (2023) 227–232
https://doi.org/10.1016/j.thorsurg.2023.04.013

which carry their own set of risks, such as hemorrhage, pneumothorax, and air embolisms.[10] All of these techniques rely on prior knowledge of the target area of interest, which is often the main limitation, particularly in cases of multiple primary tumors or metastatic disease. Delayed intraoperative identification of synchronous lesions exacerbates known poor outcomes.[11] These lesions are then also difficult to identify on subsequent surveillance computed tomographic scans owing to confounding from scar tissue adhesions, postoperative atelectasis, and lung retraction.

The 2 innovations that have propelled the increasing study of IMI are the development of fluorescent contrast agents that specifically target tumor tissues and advanced camera systems that can detect the specified fluorescence. Fluorescent dye agents are categorized by absorption and emission wavelength: those within the visible light spectrum, 390 to 700 nm, or near infrared (NIR) seen only with specialized equipment, 700 to 900 nm. The effectiveness of dye agents within 390 to 700 nm is limited, as they have poor tissue penetration secondary to scatter and absorption from surrounding light.[12] Thus, attention in IMI advancement has been on agents within NIR fluorophores. The advantages of NIR light are increased tissue depth penetration and decreased tissue autofluorescence to further highlight the lesion in question.[13] The signal detected by the camera is quantified using the tumor-to-background ratio (TBR), which is calculated by dividing the mean fluorescence intensity (MFI) of the tumor by MFI of surrounding tissue. Within NIR fluorophores, there are currently 3 nontargeted agents that have been approved in the United States. Indocyanine green (ICG), methylene blue, and 5-aminolevulinic acid are currently used for various indications, and early NIR camera systems were first designed to work with these agents.[13] ICG was the first fluorescent dye to be tested in lung cancer pathology, and over the last decade, there has been an explosion of innovation leading to more sophisticated targeted therapy, such as EC 17 and OTL38. IMI is a novel technique at the cusp of revolutionizing outcomes in thoracic surgery, and ongoing clinical trials are paving the way for this practice change.

## DISCUSSION

### *Indocyanine Green*

ICG is a nontargeted NIR fluorophore with an emission wavelength of 785 to 800 nm that accumulates in tumor tissues at high doses owing to the enhanced permeability and retention (EPR) effect. The dye extravasates from leaky capillaries in tumor tissue and cannot escape, and the EPR concept has been supported by studies showing that lesions lacking epithelial cells are not readily identified by ICG.[14,15] As the pioneering agent, ICG is already being used extensively in a local context in lung surgery. Studies have shown success with lower doses in measuring tissue perfusion, such as determining the viability of conduits in esophagectomy and identifying intersegmental planes in segmentectomy. One of the advantages of ICG is that it can be administered intravenously with limited adverse effects.

The Singhal research group has paved the way for many landmark ICG trials. Jiang and colleagues[16] performed a study determining the optimal timing and dose of ICG for IMI, which was concluded to be 5 mg/kg 24 hours before surgery. These results were used in a subsequent study by the Singhal group that identified 16 out 18 pulmonary nodules using ICG, as well as 5 additional nodules not previously identified on preoperative imaging.[15] The mean TBR was 2.2, but unfortunately the depth of penetration was limited at 1.3 cm from pleural surface, and there was significant background noise from chronic lung disease present in trial patients. This lack of discrimination between tumor tissues and the surrounding inflammatory changes was further assessed in small trial of 5 patients by Singhal and colleagues looking at tumor fluorescence ex vivo.[17] They demonstrated that in cases of mass effect from tumors where the vascular supply is threatened and there is subsequent congestion and edema, ICG and NIR imaging were unable to distinguish tumor from atelectasis and inflammation.

Mao and colleagues[18] later enrolled 36 patients into a study using the same ICG dosing and identified 68 of 76 nodules in vivo, including nodules as small as 1 mm. However, the depth of penetration was again limited at 1.3 cm from the pleural surface. Kim and colleagues[19] used a smaller dose of ICG at 1 mg/kg 24 hours preoperatively and measured fluorescence signals on the back table, which revealed 2 important findings. One, areas of obstructive pneumonia without evidence of malignancy contributed to rates of false positivity; two, MFI was not associated with tumor size or PET avidity, but with tumor depth.

Although ICG continues to be a helpful tool, its limitations cannot be ignored. Various clinical trials by Singhal, Mao, and Kim and colleagues have demonstrated consensus that ICG has limited depth penetration of approximately 1.3 cm from the pleural surface and a lack of specificity to tumor tissue.[18,19] With the discovery of these aforementioned shortcomings, research turned toward developing targeted agents.

## EC 17

Targeted agents in lung cancer were born with the discovery of a high prevalence of folate receptor-α (FRα) expression in 80% of pulmonary adenocarcinomas and 20% to 40% of squamous cell carcinomas.[20] FRα-targeted probes were already being tested in other malignancies, such as ovarian, colorectal, and head and neck cancer.[21–24] For non–small cell lung cancer, FRα expression is a positive prognostic factor and is expressed at $10^3$ to $10^4$ receptors per cell in pulmonary adenocarcinomas.[15] One of the first of these FRα-targeted agents to be studied in clinical trials was EC 17.

The Singhal group used EC 17 infusions of 0.1 mg/kg 4 hours before diagnostic wedge resection in 30 patients and identified 19 out of 19 pulmonary adenocarcinomas on ex vivo IMI.[25] This proved more accurate than frozen section analysis, which only identified 13 of the 19 nodules as adenocarcinoma. This optical biopsy technique was also more efficient, taking on average 2.4 minutes versus 26.5 minutes for frozen analysis. In a second trial, Singhal and colleagues studied 50 patients who underwent surgery with EC 17 and found that 92% of the tumors fluoresced intraoperatively, and more impressively, 2 patients were upstaged owing to the findings of previously unidentified nodules.[15] Later, this group also demonstrated the use of EC 17 as an intraoperative adjunct to assess surgical margins during tumor resection using both mice models and 3 pilot patients.[26]

Nevertheless, with an excitation wavelength of 520 nm versus ICG at 785 to 800 nm, EC 17 showed limitations in tissue penetration.[6] Tumors that fluoresced with EC 17 were shown to be much brighter ex vivo than in vivo, not owing to a change in TBR but to the additional dissection performed and more direct exposure to the camera in an ex vivo setting.[15] Although EC 17 proved to be safe, cost-effective, and better than ICG at distinguishing peritumoral inflammation and atelectasis, surgeons and scientists understood the need for advances in FRα-targeted probes.

## OTL38

As strengths and limitations were identified through trials with ICG and EC 17, an NIR and FRα-targeted probe called pafolacianine, or OTL38, was developed and approved by the Food and Drug Administration in late 2022. As opposed to EC 17, which was a short-wavelength folate-fluorescein, OTL38 was a long-wavelength tracer with emissions of approximately 793 nm. OTL38 exhibited molecular and clinical advantages, such as rapid plasma clearance and long residence time in tumors, which allowed it to be administered on the day of surgery as opposed to the day before, as seen with ICG use.[10,20]

The Singhal group compared EC 17 with OTL 38 and determined that OTL38 performed better in penetration depth, signal-to-background ratio, and frequency of tumor and margin detection.[27] The limit in penetration depth was 1.8 cm from the pleural surface for OTL38 versus 0.3 cm for EC 17. Moreover, the signal-to-background ratio was 2.71 versus 1.73 for OTL38 and EC 17, respectively ($P<.0001$).

Soon, a multi-institutional phase 2 clinical trial was undertaken by Gangadharan and colleagues[28] to assess the efficacy of OTL38 use by measuring the occurrence of clinically significant events as defined by occurrences that modified the intended operation, identified additional cancers, or upstaged the patient's cancer. Ninety-two patients were included in the study, and OTL38 performed remarkably well with the finding of 24 additional nodules, 10% of which were found to be malignant. The use of OTL38 also assisted in identifying 12% of lesions that surgeons could not localize and revealed 9% of positive resection margins that surgeons would have otherwise thought negative. The drug-related toxicities reported were few and resolved with conservative measures, and surgeons reported ease of use after just 10 cases. Patients undergoing sublobar resection received the greatest benefit with 31% of patients having a clinically significant event as opposed to 18% in lobectomy patients.

With recent publications purporting segmentectomy instead of lobectomy as the new gold standard for early-stage non–small cell lung cancer treatment, the use of IMI for precise localization and resection of small tumors proves more important than ever.[1,2] The ELUDICATE trial is a phase 3 randomized controlled trial that just completed accrual at 140 patients with the study aim of investigating the number of clinically significant events in the OTL38 arm versus the placebo arm. The results will shed light on clinical ramifications of this technology, and thoracic surgeons eagerly await the evidence that could lead to an important practice change.

## Antibody-Targeted Agents

Despite exponential growth in the field of IMI over the last decade, there are still large cohorts of patients who do not harbor FRα-positive tumors and who thus lack access to this technology. Other receptors, such as carcinoembryonic antigen (CEA) and epidermal growth factor receptor (EGFR), are known to be highly expressed in lung cancers and have become areas of potential scientific exploration.

CEA cell adhesion molecule 5 is unique, as it is expressed both on lung adenocarcinomas and in patient serum through glycoprotein detection.[29] It serves as a prognostic tool in lung adenocarcinoma and can be used in the preoperative setting to assess receptor expression through blood tests rather than invasive biopsies. The CEA antibody-targeted NIR tracer known as SGM-101 has been successfully studied in gastrointestinal adenocarcinomas, but no clinical studies to date have been conducted in lung cancer. Singhal and colleagues conducted an experiment using SGM-101 in lung adenocarcinoma using colorectal cell lines as positive controls and mesothelioma cell lines as negative controls.[29] They found that lung adenocarcinoma cell lines fluoresced with a median TBR of 3.04 versus 4.11 for the colorectal lines, whereas the mesothelioma cell lines did not fluoresce at all ($P<.05$). These preliminary results show promise for future investigations in both primary lung adenocarcinomas and pulmonary metastases from primary colorectal cancers.

On the other hand, the EGFR antibody, panitumumab, and associated NIR dye, IRDye800, have been explored in head and neck cancer as an intraoperative adjunct for assessing margin and lymph node status.[30–32] EGFR is often overexpressed in lung cancer, making it another potential target for IMI development, and a phase 1 clinical trial is currently underway. Antibody-based imaging targets also come with several advantages, including low-toxicity profiles and more specificity in targeting tumor cells.[33]

## SUMMARY

IMI is a novel and exponentially growing technology that has the ability to improve surgical and survival outcomes through precise oncologic resections. The advancements in imaging agents started with nontargeted, NIR agents (ICG), to targeted but not NIR agents (EC 17), targeted and NIR agents (OTL38), and now even to antibody-based agents. With the increasing use of minimally invasive techniques and lung preservation strategies, IMI will continue to be an important tool for tumor localization and margin assessment. With depth of tissue penetration as a persistent limitation, a new molecular imaging technique called photoacoustic imaging is now under investigation.[10,34,35] This technology overcomes the high degree of scattering of optical photons in tissue and is thus able to localize pulmonary nodules up to 7 cm from the pleural surface in preclinical studies. Ongoing work will reveal its true clinical significance, and it is hoped that alterations to fluorochromes in contrast agents will also improve tissue penetration. Future work will need to focus on enhancing IMI value in patients with chronic lung disease and significant smoking history, as studies have shown markedly decreased efficacy secondary to light-absorbing carbon deposition.[36] Last, additional targeted dyes will need to be developed to incorporate other histologies and broaden the use of IMI to all lung cancer diseases.

## CLINICS CARE POINTS

- Intraoperative molecular imaging has the potential to improve surgical management of lung cancer, particularly in identifying small tumors during sublobar resection.
- Developing targeted, near-infrared agents and fluorescence cameras will be key.
- Clinical trials are needed to ensure accuracy in intraoperative molecular imaging and to explore other uses, such as identifying additional tumors.

## DISCLOSURE

L.-Y. Wong has no disclosures. N.S. Lui has a research grant from the Intuitive Foundation, United States and Centese. She is a data safety monitor for Intuitive Surgical.

## REFERENCES

1. Saji H, Okada M, Tsuboi M, et al. West Japan Oncology Group and Japan Clinical Oncology Group. Segmentectomy versus lobectomy in small-sized peripheral non-small-cell lung cancer (JCOG0802/WJOG4607L): a multicentre, open-label, phase 3, randomised, controlled, non-inferiority trial. Lancet 2022;399(10335):1607–17.
2. Altorki NK, Wang X, Wigle D, et al. Perioperative mortality and morbidity after sublobar versus lobar resection for early-stage non-small-cell lung cancer: post-hoc analysis of an international, randomised, phase 3 trial (CALGB/Alliance 140503). Lancet Respir Med 2018;6(12):915–24.
3. Samson P, Guitron J, Reed MF, et al. Predictors of conversion to thoracotomy for video-assisted thoracoscopic lobectomy: a retrospective analysis and the influence of computed tomography-based

calcification assessment. J Thorac Cardiovasc Surg 2013;145:1512–8.
4. Sawada S, Komori E, Yamashita M. Evaluation of video-assisted thoracoscopic surgery lobectomy requiring emergency conversion to thoracotomy. Eur J Cardio Thorac Surg 2009;36:487–90.
5. Gazala S, Hunt I, Valji A, et al. A method of assessing reasons for conversion during video-assisted thoracoscopic lobectomy. Interact Cardiovasc Thorac Surg 2011;12:962–4.
6. Newton AD, Kennedy GT, Predina JD, et al. Intraoperative molecular imaging to identify lung adenocarcinomas. J Thorac Dis 2016;8(Suppl 9): S697–704.
7. Hancock JG, Rosen JE, Antonicelli A, et al. Impact of adjuvant treatment for microscopic residual disease after non-small cell lung cancer surgery. Ann Thorac Surg 2015;99:406–13.
8. Osarogiagbon RU, Ray MA, Faris NR, et al. Prognostic value of National Comprehensive Cancer Network lung cancer resection quality criteria. Ann Thorac Surg 2017;103:1557–65.
9. Tringale KR, Pang J, Nguyen QT. Image-guided surgery in cancer: a strategy to reduce incidence of positive surgical margins. Wiley Interdiscip Rev Syst Biol Med 2018;10:e1412.
10. Neijenhuis LKA, de Myunck LDAN, Bijlstra OD, et al. Near-Infrared Fluorescence Tumor-Targeted Imaging in Lung Cancer: A Systematic Review. Life 2022;12(3):446.
11. Cheng H, Lei BF, Peng PJ, et al. Histologic lung cancer subtype differentiates synchronous multiple primary lung adenocarcinomas from intrapulmonary metastases. J Surg Res 2017;211:215–22.
12. Jacques SL. Optical properties of biological tissues: a review. Phys Med Biol 2013;58:R37–61.
13. Gioux S, Choi HS, Frangioni JV. Image-guided surgery using invisible near-infrared light: fundamentals of clinical translation. Mol Imaging 2010;9:237–55.
14. Greish K. Enhanced permeability and retention of macromolecular drugs in solid tumors: a royal gate for targeted anticancer nanomedicines. J Drug Target 2007;15:457–64.
15. Okusanya OT, Holt D, Heitjan D, et al. Intraoperative near-infrared imaging can identify pulmonary nodules. Ann Thorac Surg 2014;98:1223–30.
16. Jiang JX, Keating JJ, Jesus EM, et al. Optimization of the enhanced permeability and retention effect for near-infrared imaging of solid tumors with indocyanine green. Am J Nucl Med Mol Imaging 2015;5: 390–400.
17. Holt D, Okusanya O, Judy R, et al. Intraoperative Near-Infrared Imaging Can Distinguish Cancer from Normal Tissue but Not Inflammation. Multhoff G, editor. PLoS One 2014;9(7):e103342.
18. Mao Y, Chi C, Yang F, et al. The identification of subcentimetre nodules by near-infrared fluorescence thoracoscopic systems in pulmonary resection surgeries. Eur J Cardio Thorac Surg 2017;52(6): 1190–6.
19. Kim HK, Quan YH, Choi BH, et al. Intraoperative pulmonary neoplasm identification using near-infrared fluorescence imaging. Eur J Cardio Thorac Surg 2016;49(5):1497–502.
20. Rogalla S, Joosten SCM, Alam IS, et al. Intraoperative Molecular Imaging in Lung Cancer: The State of the Art and the Future. Mol Ther 2018;26(2): 338–41.
21. Predina JD, Newton AD, Connolly C, et al. Identification of a folate receptor-targeted near-infrared molecular contrast agent to localize pulmonary adenocarcinomas. Mol Ther 2018;26:390–403. this issue.
22. Hoogstins CE, Tummers QR, Gaarenstroom KN, et al. A novel tumor-specific agent for intraoperative near-infrared fluorescence imaging: a translational study in healthy volunteers and patients with ovarian cancer. Clin Cancer Res 2016;22:2929–38.
23. Rosenthal EL, Warram JM, de Boer E, et al. Safety and tumor specificity of cetuximab-IRDye800 for surgical navigation in head and neck cancer. Clin Cancer Res 2015;21:3658–66.
24. Harlaar NJ, Koller M, de Jongh SJ, et al. Molecular fluorescence-guided surgery of peritoneal carcinomatosis of colorectal origin: a single-centre feasibility study. Lancet Gastroenterol Hepatol 2016;1: 283–90.
25. Kennedy GT, Okusanya OT, Keating JJ, et al. The optical biopsy: A novel technique for rapid intraoperative diagnosis of primary pulmonary adenocarcinomas. Ann Surg 2015;262:602–9.
26. Keating JJ, Okusanya OT, De Jesus E, et al. Intraoperative molecular imaging of lung adenocarcinoma can identify residual tumor cells at the surgical margins. Mol Imag Biol 2016;18:209–18.
27. Kennedy GT, Azari FS, Chang A, et al. Comparative Experience of Short-wavelength Versus Long-wavelength Fluorophores for Intraoperative Molecular Imaging of Lung Cancer. Ann Surg 2022;276(4): 711–9.
28. Gangadharan S, Sarkaria IN, Rice D, et al. Multiinstitutional Phase 2 Clinical Trial of Intraoperative Molecular Imaging of Lung Cancer. Ann Thorac Surg 2021;112(4):1150–9.
29. Azari F, Kennedy GT, Chang A, et al. Glycoprotein Receptor CEACAM5-Targeted Intraoperative Molecular Imaging Tracer in Non-Small Cell Lung Cancer. Ann Thorac Surg 2022. https://doi.org/10.1016/j.athoracsur.2022.05.019. S0003-4975(22)00731-00737.
30. Fakurnejad S, Krishnan G, van Keulen S, et al. Intraoperative Molecular Imaging for ex vivo Assessment of Peripheral Margins in Oral Squamous Cell Carcinoma. Front Oncol 2019;9:1476.

31. Van Keulen S, van den Berg NS, Nishio N, et al. Rapid, non-invasive fluorescence margin assessment: Optical specimen mapping in oral squamous cell carcinoma. Oral Oncol 2019;88:58–65.
32. Nishio N, van den Berg NS, van Keulen S, et al. Optical molecular imaging can differentiate metastatic from benign lymph nodes in head and neck cancer. Nat Commun 2019 06;10(1):5044.
33. Warram JM, de Boer E, Sorace AG, et al. Antibody-based imaging strategies for cancer. Cancer Metastasis Rev 2014;33(2–3):809–22.
34. Wang LV, Hu S. Photoacoustic Tomography: In Vivo Imaging from Organelles to Organs. Science 2012; 335:1458–62.
35. Lee CY, Fujino K, Motooka Y, et al. Photoacoustic imaging to localize indeterminate pulmonary nodules: A preclinical study. PLoS One 2020;15:e0231488.
36. Azari F, Kennedy G, Zhang K, et al. Effects of Light-absorbing Carbons in Intraoperative Molecular Imaging-Guided Lung Cancer Resections. Mol Imaging Biol 2022. https://doi.org/10.1007/s11307-021-01699-6.

# Single Setting Robotic Lung Nodule Diagnosis and Resection

Priya P. Patel, MD, DAABIP[a,*], Duy Kevin Duong, DO, DAABIP[a], Amit K. Mahajan, MD, FCCP, DAABIP[a], Taryne A. Imai, MD, MEHP[b]

**KEYWORDS**

• Bronchoscopy • Lung cancer • Lobectomy • Lung nodule • Resection • Robotic

**KEY POINTS**

- Robotic-assisted bronchoscopy improves reach, stability, and precision in the field of bronchoscopic lung nodule biopsy.
- Robotic-assisted lung surgery have shown to improve short-term perioperative outcomes and similar long-term oncologic outcomes and hospital costs compared with traditional lung surgery.
- Combining lung cancer diagnostics with therapeutic surgical resection into a single-setting anesthesia procedure has potential to decrease costs, improve patient experience, and reduce delays in cancer care.

## INTRODUCTION

Lung cancer is among the most frequently diagnosed cancers globally, accounting for 2.2 million new cases in 2020.[1] It is the leading cause of cancer-related deaths in the United States and worldwide with an estimated 1.7 million deaths annually.[2,3] The overall 5-year survival for lung cancer is currently 21%, lower than many other leading cancer sites such as colorectal (65%), breast (89.6%), and prostate (98.2%).[4,5] Due to advances in lung cancer detection and implementation of screening programs in high-risk individuals, the frequency of locally advanced disease amenable to a curative intent therapy has increased. Although only accounting for 16% of newly diagnosed lung cancer cases, the 5-year survival for early-stage (stage I and II) lung cancer is 56%.[2,4–6]

The initial management of patients with lung cancer depends heavily on the type of lung cancer and the extent of its involvement. Non-small-cell lung cancers (NSCLCs) account for approximately 85% of all new lung cancer diagnoses, with small-cell lung cancer (SCLC) making up the remaining.[7] For early stage or locally advanced diseases, the preferred definitive treatment is surgical resection of the tumor. Surgical resection provides the best opportunity for long-term survival and cure in patients, with recent studies showing overall survival of Stage IA1-IA2 to be 92% to 83% at 5 years.[4–6]

Historically, the challenge has been timely detection of lung cancer. This is largely because patients are typically asymptomatic when the disease is at an early stage. There were 240,000 new lung cancers diagnosed in the United States (U.S.) in 2020, approximately 70% of which presented with advanced local or metastatic disease not amenable to cure.[5]

Fortunately, a landmark study entitled the National Lung Screening Trial (NLST) demonstrated a 20% reduction in mortality from lung cancer screening using low-dose computed tomography (LDCT) screening of high-risk individuals.[8] This subsequently led to the United States Preventive

[a] Interventional Pulmonology, Inova Health System, Schar Cancer Institute, 8081 Innovation Park Drive, Suite 3000, Fairfax, VA 22031, USA; [b] The Queen's University Medical Group, Queen's Health System, University of Hawaii, 1356 Lusitana Street, 6th floor, Honolulu, HI 96813, USA
* Corresponding author.
*E-mail address:* Priya.patel2@inova.org

Thorac Surg Clin 33 (2023) 233–244
https://doi.org/10.1016/j.thorsurg.2023.04.009
1547-4127/23/

Services Task Force (USPSTF) recommending annual screening of high-risk persons.[9] Since then, there has been an increase in establishment of lung cancer screening programs worldwide. This along with the increasing availability of CT has led to a predicted 1.6 million new pulmonary nodules to be detected in the U.S. annually.[10] Although the majority of these nodules may require only surveillance imaging, many will require biopsy. The NLST and similar trials (ie, NELSON) showed that most nodules detected (~80%) were located in the periphery of the lung.[8,11] This presents a new set of challenges in relation to both safely diagnosing these often small peripheral lung nodules as well as subsequently identifying these nodules intraoperatively for surgical resection.

One of the biggest challenges in lung cancer management is minimizing the time from diagnosis to therapeutic treatment. Treatment delays, defined as resection 8 weeks or more after diagnosis, are more likely to be upstaged, have increased 30-day mortality, and decreased median survival.[12] In addition, these delays have been found on retrospective analysis to be associated with higher costs.[13] Patients can experience long periods of delay between their first diagnostic test for lung cancer and a definitive diagnosis, with 46% of lung cancer patients requiring two or more biopsies. In these cases, surgical biopsy with wedge resection can be directly indicated, despite being a more invasive option, with an associated 10% to 20% benign resection rate.[14] These delays can lead to more advanced stages at the time of diagnosis, which then contribute to higher costs.[13] Therefore, the ability to combine procedures that diagnose and treat early-stage lung cancer may allow for less resource utilization and costs. Here, we present an innovative pathway to expedite lung cancer care, performing a robot-assisted navigational bronchoscopy (RAB) for diagnosis, mediastinal staging when applicable, and robot-assisted thoracoscopic surgery (RATS) for definitive treatment under a single-setting anesthesia event.

In this editorial, we intend to focus on robotic-assisted bronchoscopy (RAB) and robotic-assisted thoracoscopic surgery (RATS). This review is broadly divided into the following major sections.

1. Lung cancer diagnostics: robotic-assisted bronchoscopy
2. Lung cancer resection: robotic-assisted thoracoscopic surgery
3. Single-setting anesthesia event
    a. Preoperative evaluation
    b. Intraoperative methods
        i. RAB
        ii. RATS
4. Ongoing studies
5. Conclusion

## LUNG CANCER DIAGNOSTICS

The American College of Chest Physicians and National Comprehensive Cancer Network guidelines recommend diagnosis of the primary lesion, staging, and obtaining tissue for molecular testing using the least invasive modality and ideally in a single procedure.[15,16] An initial bronchoscopic approach for many patients facilitates both biopsies of the primary lesion and mediastinal staging before a curative-intent therapy if an option. The set of tools that allow for navigation, confirmation of target proximity, and acquisition of tissue is collectively known as guided bronchoscopy.[17] The main components of guided bronchoscopy are image-based airway navigation, real-time airway visualization, intraoperative confirmatory imaging, and specimen-acquisition tools. Fundamental prospective trials have elucidated the strengths and weaknesses of guided bronchoscopy.[18–25] These studies defined diagnostic yield, evaluated safety data, and compared guided bronchoscopy methods with percutaneous sampling, consistently finding it to be safer relative to transthoracic sampling.[26,27] Unfortunately, the diagnostic yield of guided bronchoscopy has been inconsistent in randomized controlled trials, ranging from 44% to 74%, compared with rates above 90% for percutaneous sampling.[19–27]

To overcome these limitations, robotic-assisted bronchoscopy (RAB) platforms were developed and approved by the Food and Drug Administration (FDA).[28,29] The Ion Robotic-Assisted Endoluminal Platform (Intuitive Surgical, Inc.) is based on the novel shape-sensing RAB (ssRAB) technology (**Fig. 1**).[30,31] The Monarch RAB platform (Auris Health, Inc.) is based on electromagnetic navigation (EMN RAB) technology.[32] RAB is designed to allow endobronchial navigation into the lung periphery while allowing direct visualization of peripheral airways and maintaining catheter stability and shape to maximize precision during sampling (**Fig. 2**). These advantages of RAB have been previously demonstrated in cadaveric models and subsequently in several pivotal studies demonstrating a navigational success rate between 96.2% and 100%.[33–40] Diagnostic yield for malignancy was found to be 69.1% using EMN RAB and as high as 88% using ssRAB.[33–39] Large-volume studies evaluating diagnostic yield remain scarce; however, such studies are being initiated widely given the widespread adoption and use of RAB. There is consistent evidence to show that with RAB, reach, stability, and precision are no

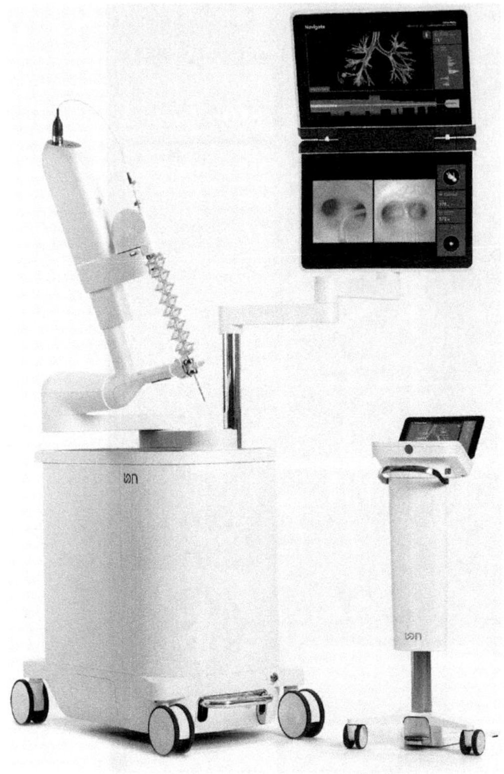

Fig. 1. Ion robotic-assisted endoluminal platform. (© 2023 Intuitive Surgical Operations, Inc.)

longer in question as compared to previous navigational technologies. Another benefit includes the seamless integration of RAB technology with endobronchial ultrasound (EBUS), radial EBUS, fluoroscopy, cone beam computed tomography, and the da Vinci Surgical System (Intuitive Surgical, Inc., **Fig. 3**).

Another challenge that has been improved using RAB is marking of small peripheral lung lesions. Localization of small peripheral lung lesions, solid or subsolid, can prove to be problematic for thoracic surgeons who need to localize these nonpalpable subcentimeter nodules. With the increasing adoption of the robotic platform within thoracic surgery, localization becomes more important given the loss of haptic feedback with robotic surgery. Current methods for marking lung nodules include percutaneous coils, hook-wire, or radiotracer placement by interventional radiologists using CT guidance. Although these methods have been found to be effective, the higher rate of pneumothorax, bleeding, hematoma, and dislodgement of tracer are noted limitations as compared to guided bronchoscopy.[41,42] Furthermore, these techniques require coordination between multiple specialists and often times result in significant delay to surgical resection.[41–45] Bronchoscopic lung nodule marking on the other hand has been found to be effective and safe.[46,47] The methods for localizing peripheral lung nodules using RAB include but are not limited to dye marking (using methylene blue, indocyanine green, or iopamidol) or fiducial marker placement.

### *Cost*

Hospital cost has remained one of the main limitations associated with development and integration of new technology in any hospital system. RAB platforms require initial capital investment, including purchase price of the robotic unit as well as specialized disposable supplies and maintenance. Given the recent integration of RAB, there are no studies showing costs associated with RAB. Although initial startup costs are considerable, the downstream growth of lung cancer screening programs, pulmonary nodule programs, and cancer care (medical oncology, thoracic surgery, radiation oncology referrals) result in revenue that will likely surmount these. The improved accuracy and diagnostic yield of RAB enable biopsy of smaller subcentimeter nodules, therefore decreasing the population of “watchful waiters” or patients who are receiving serial surveillance CT scans. By decreasing the watchful waiter population, RAB can offer less CT scans, reduced resource utilization, and most importantly peace of mind to patients with a benign diagnosis or can now minimize further delays and initiate plans for staging and surgery for those patients diagnosed with malignancy. Further studies showing cost of integration and downstream revenues are needed to further clarify this relationship.

## LUNG CANCER RESECTION

The first report of robotic-assisted thoracoscopic surgery (RATS) for anatomic lung resection was published in 2002.[48] Since the initial report, the national utilization rate of the robotic-assisted approach for lung resection has continued to increase.[49] The technical advantages of robotic technology for lung resection include high-definition three-dimensional visualization, wristed instrumentation for improved maneuverability with 7° of freedom, tremor filtration, and improved lymph node sampling.[50–52] In recent published data, robotic-assisted lobectomies have shown improved short-term perioperative outcomes and similar long-term oncologic outcomes and hospital costs compared with traditional open thoracotomy or video-assisted thoracoscopy.[53,54] Furthermore, higher volume centers with established expertise have showed lower conversion rates and improved perioperative outcomes.[55] Merritt and colleagues

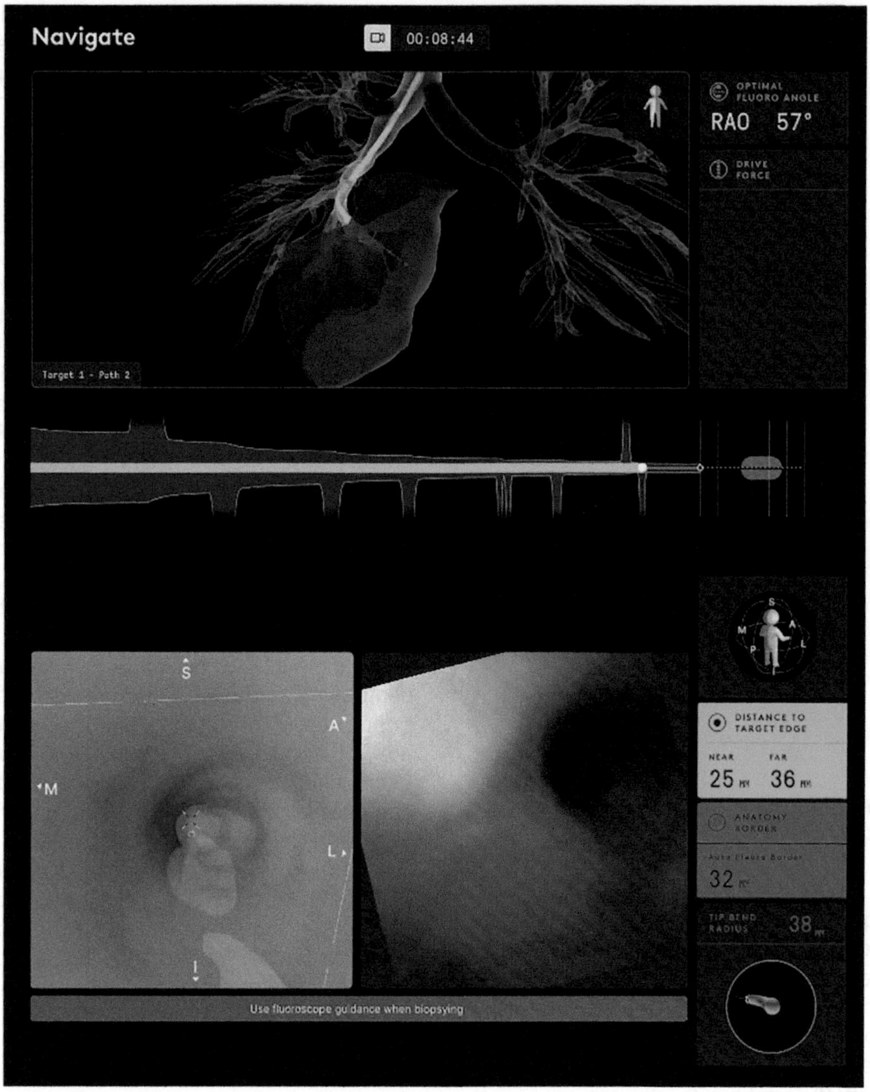


**Fig. 2.** Robotic assisted bronchoscopy is designed to allow endobronchial navigation into the lung periphery while allowing direct visualization of peripheral airways and maintaining catheter stability and shape to maximize precision during sampling.

reviewed temporal changes in case volume, costs, and postoperative outcomes for RATS in 1001 cases, between 2009 and 2021.[56] The overall postoperative complication rate decreased from 46.1% (first 500 cases) to 29.6% for second 500 cases ($P < .0001$). The median hospital stay decreased from 4 days to 3 days ($P < .0001$). They concluded that with increasing institutional experience, perioperative outcomes may continuously improve in RATS.[56]

Advantages of the robotic platform have also facilitated performing parenchymal sparing anatomic resections. Segmentectomy, as a surgical resection option for the treatment of NSCLC, is a more technically demanding operation than lobectomy and requires familiarity of the segmental anatomy. Although a minimally invasive approach, video-assisted thoracoscopic surgery (VATS) is limited when performing segmentectomies because of its 2-dimensional visualization and use of rigid instruments that restrict maneuverability in the chest. These limitations present challenges when performing the distal dissection and isolation of segmental vessels and bronchi that are required to perform a segmentectomy. Features of the robotic platform may mitigate these technical demands. Furthermore, with increased utilization of lung cancer screening and the ability of RAB to accurately diagnose cancer within small subcentimeter pulmonary nodules, the gold standard treatment of performing

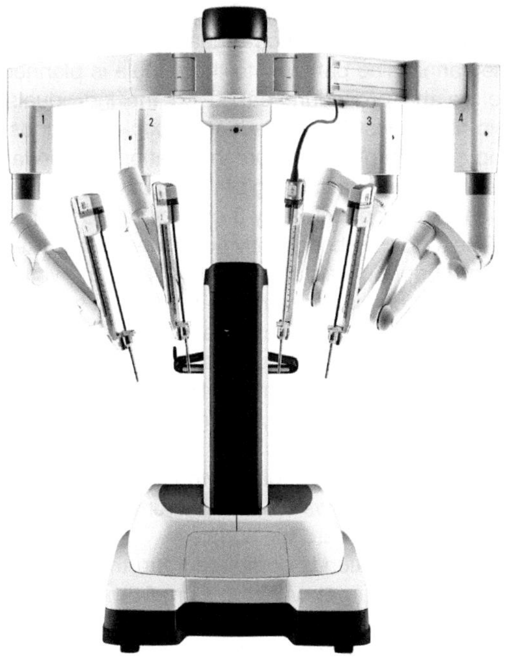


**Fig. 3.** Da Vinci surgical system, Xi. (© 2023 Intuitive Surgical Operations, Inc.)

lobectomies may unnecessarily resect healthy parenchyma. Therefore, increased application of RAB may increase the number of segmentectomies being performed. Many have already supported and proven equivalent short-term perioperative outcomes and long-term survival between segmentectomy and lobectomy in patients with clinical stage T1a NSCLC, which may further increase adoption of robotic surgery and segmentectomy.[57,58]

### *Cost*

One of the main limitations associated with the use of robotic surgery platforms is the associated hospital costs. Robotic surgery specific costs include the instruments (each with limited number of uses), the specialized disposable supplies, the capital investment (including purchase price of the robotic unit), and the ongoing maintenance fees. Unlike RAB which is a newer technology, in current literature, hospital costs associated with RATS vary greatly among studies. A frequent finding across several studies has shown that approximately half of the total hospital costs related to RATS are incurred in the postoperative setting, with postoperative complications and prolonged hospital stays adding considerable expenses.[53,59,60] One such study supports this; Merritt and colleagues demonstrated a significant decrease in median direct and indirect hospital costs, as well as decreased median direct and indirect operating room costs over time for RATS. This observed decrease was thought to be due to concomitant decrease in hospital length of stay, postoperative complications, and admissions to the intensive care unit.[56] Several studies have also found that although the cost of RATS is still higher than that of VATS, it is typically equal or lower to that of traditional open lobectomy.[61,62] There is also evidence supporting high-volume centers can operate at a lower per-procedure cost. At high-volume centers, the total cost of RATS lobectomy was the lowest (in comparison to VATS and open thoracotomy).[61,62]

## SINGLE SETTING ANESTHESIA EVENT

### *Preoperative Evaluation*

A thin slice (1.0-mm slices) chest CT imaging is obtained for preprocedural planning and staging purposes. A positron emission tomography (PET) is used for further risk classification of the lung nodule in question, evaluation of the N2 lymph nodes, and to assess for distant metastatic disease. During preoperative medical and surgical evaluation, pulmonary function testing is obtained to evaluate permissibility and appropriateness of surgical resection (ie, segmentectomy or lobectomy). Further testing is completed as indicated or appropriate in surgical planning, that is, ventilation/perfusion imaging or cardiac evaluation. The patient is consented for both the RAB and RATS (in case if malignancy is confirmed on examination intraoperatively). Both procedures will be completed under a single anesthesia event.

### *Preoperative Selection*

Patient selection for the single anesthetic pathway is integral for various reasons, including optimizing operating room block time, minimizing the occult N2 disease rate, and limiting benign resections. Although no published criteria exist for the single anesthetic pathway of lung cancer care, the following are criteria our program follows.

- Nodule suspicious for NSCLC (smoking history, upper lobe location, spiculated, increasing in size)
- Nodule size less than 3 cm
- No chest wall or surrounding structure invasion
- No mediastinal adenopathy
- No PET avidity in the mediastinum
- Clinical stage 1 to 2 NSCLC (avoid high probability of N2 disease patients)
- Moderate to excellent PFTs with good performance status

- Patients who travel from far distance to receive treatment
- Agreeable and trusting patient personality

### Team Training and Preparation

A single anesthetic pathway to lung cancer care is a multidisciplinary endeavor, requiring collaboration and cooperation from many service lines. Discussions with radiology involve performing CT scans using robotic navigational bronchoscopy protocols with the appropriate slice thickness and amount of overlap. Working with pathology involves a shift in perspective for fine-needle aspiration (FNA) specimens, as cytologist not only have to make intraoperative judgements on tissue adequacy but also provide a diagnosis of malignancy or benign. Furthermore, discussion regarding workflows between the proceduralist and the pathologists is important to optimize efficiency and minimize the burden of processing multiple cytology and frozen section specimens. The anesthesia team are integral participants in the single anesthetic pathway and workflows. Discussion regarding, intubation strategies (single lumen transition to double lumen), ventilator settings, and timing of line placements are important to have before the procedure. Furthermore, operating room staff training is necessary to ensure safe and efficient procedures. As multiple machines (RAB platform, C-arm, EBUS, DaVinci patient cart, and console) are required for a single anesthetic setting, the operating room can become very crowded. Dry runs practicing moving the machines in and out of the operating room safely, timing of procedure setup, and patient positioning optimize success of the procedures.

The workflow and division of labor between the interventional pulmonologist and thoracic surgeon can have various permutations. The pulmonologist may first perform the RAB biopsy and EBUS, then the surgeon performs the robotic resection. In some cases, the surgeon may perform all stages (biopsy, mediastinal staging, and resection) of a single anesthetic event. Some have done RAB biopsy and EBUS in a bronchoscopy or endoscopy suite and then move the patient to the operating room for resection, while most will perform all stages of the single anesthetic event in the operating room.

Workflow and landscape of the single anesthetic procedure is individualized by institution and dependent on the resources present.

### Intraoperative Methods

Part I: RAB—Diagnosis with confirmation ± marking.

For robotic bronchoscopy, the patient is placed under general anesthesia with paralysis in the supine position. A single-lumen endotracheal tube (ETT) is used, at least size 8, and positioned under bronchoscopic guidance at least 2 to 3 cm from the carina. The pathway to the nodule is planned before the procedure based on the individuals' thin-slice chest CT. A standard flexible bronchoscopy is completed before navigation for airway clearance and positioning of the tip of the endotracheal tube approximately 3 cm above the carina.

The robot is subsequently positioned and docked to an endotracheal tube adapter. Next, the virtual bronchoscopy is registered to the patient's airway in real time. The main carina is marked for orientation. Each lobe of the lung is then registered by driving into each subsegment of the upper and lower lobes. After registration, navigation begins using real-time bronchoscopic view of the patient's airways complemented with a virtual bronchoscopy image, which shows a "cookie-crumb" path as a guide to drive toward the nodule.

Once navigation is completed and the lesion of interest is in target within 1-3 cm from the tip of the catheter, the vision probe is removed (when using the Ion Endoluminal System), and a radial endobronchial ultrasound (R-EBUS) is used to detect a signal coinciding with the lesion. Sometimes, when biopsy requires traversing a cartilaginous bronchial wall, a needle is used to puncture the wall to create a path for the R-EBUS probe to pass through to confirm the location of the lesion. Once confirmed, biopsies are taken under image guidance with a variety of available adjunct imaging platforms such as 2D fluoroscopy, 3D fluoroscopy, or cone-beam CT scan. Biopsies tools, which include flexible needles of various sizes for FNA samples and forceps for frozen-section specimens, are passed through the catheter. Cytology slides from FNA samples can be read with rapid on-site pathologic examination (ROSE) in the most efficient setting. However, ROSE is not a requirement, and many institutions have developed pathways without ROSE capabilities. Forceps specimens can be processed by frozen section for intraoperative interpretation or by touch-prep and cytologic interpretation.

Once a diagnosis of malignancy is confirmed, the proceduralist has the option to place fiducial markers or inject dye to mark the location of the nodule. One option for dye marking, uses a mixture of 0.5 mL of methylene blue and 0.5 mL of ICG. The 1.0-mL total volume includes priming of the needle, and it is not necessary to clear the needle with air. This prevents spraying of the dye and maximizes the concentration of the dye at the site of the lesion. These adjunctive tools can greatly facilitate robotic surgical resection as lesion localization depends on visual cues and not haptic feedback. Furthermore, utilization of dye marking is most impactful when

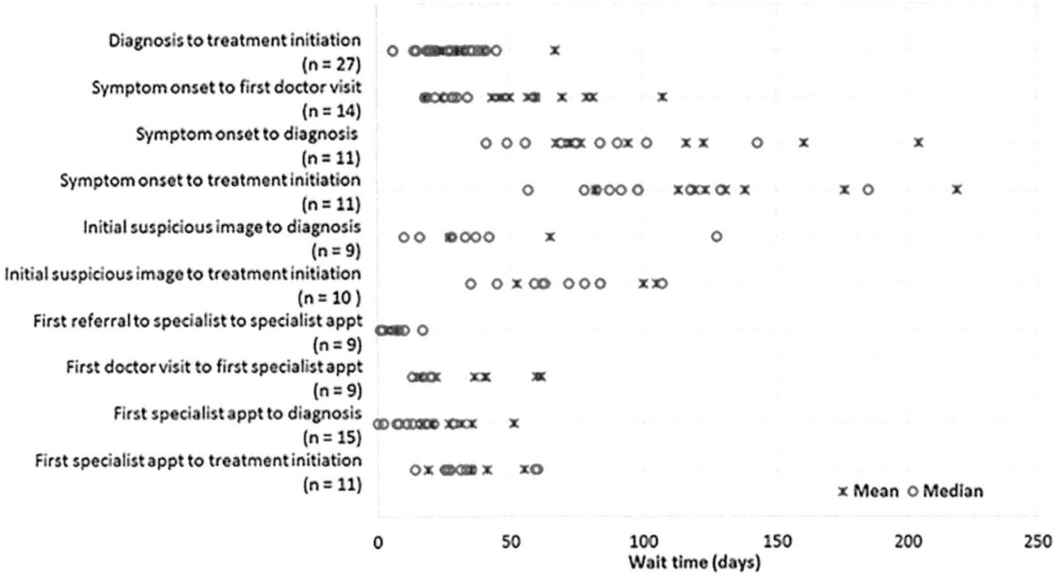


**Fig. 4.** Wait Times Experienced by Patients Along the Lung Cancer Care Continuum. Wait times reported in the literature for the ten most frequent intervals are plotted. Wait-time intervals and the total number of articles (*N*) reporting the interval are provided on the y-axis and wait time in days is on the x-axis. Stars indicate mean values and circles indicate median values. Some articles report both mean and median. Patients are experiencing a wide range of wait times for lung cancer care. Appt: appointment. (*From* Jacobsen MM, Silverstein SC, Quinn M, et al. Timeliness of access to lung cancer diagnosis and treatment: A scoping literature review. Lung Cancer. 2017;112:156-164.)

performing segmentectomies to confirm appropriate segmental location, which avoids unnecessary parenchymal resection, ensures adequate margins, and allows for efficient resection by providing intraoperative visualization of the lesion.[63]

Thereafter, the optical probe is then inserted again through the catheter to confirm adequate hemostasis. The robotic bronchoscope is then withdrawn and undocked from the ETT.

*Mediastinal staging.*

Mediastinal staging, if applicable, is then performed according to the standard oncologic guidelines. Most frequently, staging is performed with EBUS and sampling of N2 lymph nodes. ROSE or intraoperative cytology interpretation then confirms the absence or presence of metastatic malignant disease.

If the nodule biopsy confirms malignancy and mediastinal staging examination is negative for N2 metastatic disease, the patient directly undergoes RATS for surgical treatment of their lung cancer.

Part II: RATS.

At this time, the single-lumen endotracheal tube is exchanged for a double-lumen endotracheal tube, and the patient is positioned in the lateral decubitus position. For a robotic-assisted thoracoscopic surgery for resection of malignant lung nodule, the da Vinci Surgical System (Intuitive Surgical, Inc., see **Fig. 3**) is used. The robotic surgical system is equipped with a surgeon console (surgeons view and wristed instrument control), patient cart (four instrument arms), and a vision cart (allows communication between different components of system and screen for viewability). The operative lung is isolated, and insufflation of the chest commences. Robotic ports are placed, and according to surgeon preference in the interspaces of the ribs, the robot is then docked to the ports. The most up-to-date system is the da Vinci Xi Surgical System, which allows the endoscope (camera) to be placed in any position needed and can be changed throughout the operation. Various instruments are placed in the robotic arms to perform the operation. Type of resection is dependent on size and location of the tumor and surgeon preference.

## ONGOING STUDIES

Several large centers are currently studying the benefits and outcomes of single anesthesia events for robotic assisted lung nodule diagnosis and resection. Ross and colleagues, at Mainline Health System (Philadelphia, PA), have implemented a "fast-track" pathway for patients with undiagnosed and suspicious lung nodules. Their initial evaluation included 51 patients who underwent robotic-assisted bronchoscopy, of which 11 were selected for the "fast-track" pathway. Ten of these patients had single anesthesia for robotic-assisted diagnosis and resection, and one patient was diagnosed with granulomatous disease by ROSE. Nodule localization was completed with ICG in nine patients to aid in resection. No conversions to open thoracotomy were needed. There were no complications or mortalities related to either procedure.[64] They concluded that this was a safe and effective platform to diagnose and manage pulmonary nodules. Combining the diagnosis and resection to a single anesthesia event was found to shorten the time to definitive therapy, reduce patient anxiety, and enhance patient experience all without impacting risk or hospital course. Ross and colleagues subsequently evaluated a cohort of patients who underwent robotic bronchoscopy for undiagnosed pulmonary nodules followed by robotic resection via what they coined the "MIDAS" (minimally invasive diagnosis and surgery) pathway. Using clinical history and findings, patients with nodules were stratified using a preferred algorithm to earlier resection or expectant management. Fifty-two patients were included. Surgical resection and pathology confirmed malignancy in 42 patients and benign disease in 10 patients. Robotic bronchoscopy on site cytopathology confirmed malignancy in 34 patients and was nondiagnostic in 8 patients (malignancy confirmed on surgical resection). Two patients had on site cytopathology suspicious for malignancy but were found to show benign disease on resected specimens. Benign or nonspecific disease was seen on site cytopathological evaluation with surgical resection confirmed benign disease subsequently. They concluded this approach may identify patients for whom resection is indicated in a nondiagnostic bronchoscopy setting as well as reduce the number of patients resected for benign disease.[65]

These studies are still in early stages and of smaller volume; however, they do show future promise to optimizing early-stage lung cancer management.

## SUMMARY

Timely detection, diagnosis, and subsequent treatment for lung cancer is critical to patient outcomes and well-being. Significant emotional distress, impaired quality of life, increased use of health care resources, and increased cost of care are all detrimental outcomes of delays in timely diagnosis and treatment of cancer.[66] The Institute of Medicine's Committee on Quality Health Care in America recognizes timeliness in care as 1 of 6 important dimensions of health care quality.[67] In the United States, there are no federal standardized guidelines regarding timeliness of lung cancer care. In 2000, the RAND Corporation (a research organization) following a set of recommendations set forth by the British Thoracic Society published target intervals for lung cancer access to care.[68] These recommendations advocate lung cancer diagnoses should be established within 2 months after initial abnormal imaging and treatment offered within 6 weeks after diagnosis.[68] More recently, the United Kingdom's National Optimal Lung Cancer Pathway proposed that patient assessment pathways help achieve maximum waiting times of 14 days for diagnosis and 28 days for treatment.[69,70] Unfortunately, these standards are not always upheld. Jacobsen and colleagues[71] completed a systematic review on timeliness of lung cancer care including 65 studies from across 21 countries between 2007 and 2016. This study reported a median wait time from PCP referral to specialist consultation of 1 to 17 days and range median delay from diagnosis to treatment of 6 to 45 days, with an unweighted median time to treatment of 22 days. They also estimated 15% to 63% of patients were not receiving treatment within 31 days of diagnosis (**Fig. 4**).[71] Barriers such as numerous procedures, necessary repetitious procedures, lack of appointments available for specialist visits or procedures, and delays due to physicians not initially suspecting cancer were noted among the studies included.[71] Broader reasons may include greater subspecialization in the medical field, unmet care coordination, and communication needs across specialties, as well as increasing complexity and fragmentation of care.

A potential solution to these barriers is multidisciplinary evaluation that leads to timely diagnosis and optimal treatment.[72,73] With multidisciplinary involvement, as soon as a lung cancer is suspected, effective coordination and communication for timely care is possible.[72,73] Single-setting anesthesia events that include robotic lung nodule diagnosis to immediate robotic lung resection can also help mitigate these delays. Despite being new and costly technology, the use of robot-assisted procedures has increased dramatically over the last decade. Data are continually emerging that robotic assisted procedures may also provide an upper hand in terms of lung cancer diagnostics and perioperative outcomes for surgical resection relative to previous guided bronchoscopy and VATS (or thoracotomy).[33,39,40,53–56] These technologies allow for a streamline of diagnosis, staging, and treatment for one of the most common cancers. Currently, there is a paucity of high-level evidence to establish recommendations supporting single-setting anesthesia events. However, several large centers are continuing to prove benefits, including decreasing time from diagnosis to treatment.[64,65] The following are value propositions for the single anesthetic pathway to lung cancer care.

- Shortened timeline from nodule identification to definitive therapy
- Stage shift to earlier stage and improved outcomes and survival
- Elimination of high anxiety interval between diagnosis and resection
- Enhanced patient satisfaction with a comprehensive plan
- Potential reduction in risks associated with multiple anesthetic events
- Maximize pulmonary lung sparing procedures
- Decreased impact on family resources
- Earlier return to employment and usual lifestyle
- Possible decreased cost in lung cancer care without compromising oncologic standards

Developing diagnostic pathways that enhance accuracy, limit interventions, reduce risk, and facilitate earlier diagnosis and treatment of malignancy offer patients an optimized approach for nodule management. Large, multicenter, prospective randomized controlled trials are needed to identify best practices and improve current clinical practices. Additional areas of investigation may include evaluation of patient and clinician joint decision-making processes, as well as patient reported outcomes such as quality of life, burden of healthcare costs, and fear of long-term complications.

The optimal diagnostic and resection strategy is likely one that offers a multicentric perspective, including the treating physicians, a multidisciplinary team, and most importantly, the patient. After all, the overwhelming burden of cancer diagnosis, treatment, and desire for survival lie with the patient.

## CLINICS CARE POINTS

- Overall, 5-year survival for lung cancer is currently 21%, lower than other leading cancer sites such as colorectal (65%), breast (89.6%), and prostate (98.2%).
- In United States, of new lung cancer cases diagnosed, 70% presented with advanced local or metastatic disease not amenable to cure.
- Accounting for only 16% of newly diagnosed lung cancer cases, the 5-year survival for early stage (stage I and II) lung cancer is 56%.
- Surgical resection provides the best opportunity for longterm survival and cure in patients, recent studies showing overall survival of Stage IA1-IA2 to be 92% and 83% at 5 years.
- Treatment delays, defined as resection 8 weeks or more after diagnosis, are more likely to be upstaged, have increased 30-day mortality, and decreased medial survival.
- Patients can experience prolonged periods of delay between their first diagnostic test for lung cancer and definitive diagnosis, with 46% of lung cancer patients requiring two or more biopsies.
- In these cases, surgical resection can be indicated, with an associated 10-20% benign resection rate.
- Ability to combine procedures that diagnosed and treat early-stage lung cancer may allow for less resource utilization and costs.

## ACKNOWLEDGEMENT

Cari Tomayko (Intuitive Surgical, Inc.)

## REFERENCES

1. Sung H, Ferlay J, Siegel RL, et al. Global Cancer Statistics 2020: GLOBOCAN Estimates of Incidence and Mortality Worldwide for 36 Cancers in 185 Countries. CA Cancer J Clin 2021;71(3):209–49.
2. Key Statistics About Lung Cancer. Available at: https://www.cancer.org/cancer/lung-cancer/about/key-statistics.html. Accessed December 22, 2022.
3. DeSantis CE, Lin CC, Mariotto AB, et al. Cancer treatment and survivorship statistics. CA Cancer J Clin 2014;64(4):252–71.
4. Noone AM, Howlader N, Krapcho M, et al. SEER cancer statistics review, 1975-2015. National Cancer Institute; 2016.
5. Siegel RL, Miller KD, Jemal A. Cancer statistics. CA Cancer J Clin 2020;70(1):7–30. https://doi.org/10.3322/caac.21590.
6. Latest global cancer data: Cancer burden rises to 18.1 million new cases and 9.6 million cancer deaths in 2018. International Agency for Research on Cancer. Available at: https://www.iarc.who.int/wp-content/uploads/2018/09/pr263_E.pdf. Accessed December 22, 2022.
7. Molina JR, Yang P, Cassivi SD, et al. Non-small cell lung cancer: Epidemiology, risk factors, treatment, and survivorship. Mayo Clin Proc 2008;83(5):584–94.
8. Reduced Lung-Cancer Mortality with Low-Dose Computed Tomographic Screening. N Engl J Med 2011;365(5):395–409.

9. de Koning HJ, Meza R, Plevritis SK, et al. Benefits and harms of computed tomography lung cancer screening strategies: a comparative modeling study for the U.S. Preventive Services Task Force. Ann Intern Med 2014;160(5):311–20.
10. Gould MK, Tang T, Liu I-LA, et al. Recent Trends in the Identification of Incidental Pulmonary Nodules. Am J Respir Crit Care Med 2015;192(10):1208–14.
11. Yousaf-Khan U, van der Aalst C, de Jong PA, et al. Final screening round of the NELSON lung cancer screening trial: the effect of a 2.5-year screening interval. Thorax 2017;72(1):48–56.
12. Samson P, Patel A, Garrett T, et al. Effects of Delayed Surgical Resection on Short-Term and Long-Term Outcomes in Clinical Stage I Non-Small Cell Lung Cancer. Ann Thorac Surg 2015;99(6):1906–12 [discussion: 1913].
13. Gildea TR, DaCosta Byfield S, Hogarth DK, et al. A retrospective analysis of delays in the diagnosis of lung cancer and associated costs. Clinicoecon Outcomes Res 2017;9:261–9.
14. Oudkerk M, Devaraj A, Vliegenthart R, et al. European position statement on lung cancer screening. Lancet Oncol 2017;18(12):e754–66.
15. Gould MK, Donington J, Lynch WR, et al. Evaluation of individuals with pulmonary nodules: when is it lung cancer? Diagnosis and management of lung cancer, 3rd ed: American College of Chest Physicians evidence-based clinical practice guidelines. Chest 2013;143(5 Suppl):e93S–120S.
16. Ettinger DS, Wood DE, Aisner DL, et al. NCCN Guidelines Insights: Non-Small Cell Lung Cancer, Version 2.2021. J Natl Compr Cancer Netw 2021;19(3):254–66.
17. Panchabhai TS, Mehta AC. Historical perspectives of bronchoscopy. Connecting the dots. Ann Am Thorac Soc 2015;12(5):631–41.
18. Oki M, Saka H, Ando M, et al. Ultrathin Bronchoscopy with Multimodal Devices for Peripheral Pulmonary Lesions. A Randomized Trial. Am J Respir Crit Care Med 2015;192(4):468–76.
19. Folch EE, Pritchett MA, Nead MA, et al. Electromagnetic Navigation Bronchoscopy for Peripheral Pulmonary Lesions: One-Year Results of the Prospective, Multicenter NAVIGATE Study. J Thorac Oncol Off Publ Int Assoc Study Lung Cancer 2019;14(3):445–58.
20. Gildea TR, Mazzone PJ, Karnak D, et al. Electromagnetic navigation diagnostic bronchoscopy: a prospective study. Am J Respir Crit Care Med 2006;174(9):982–9.
21. Ost DE, Ernst A, Lei X, et al. Diagnostic Yield and Complications of Bronchoscopy for Peripheral Lung Lesions. Results of the AQuIRE Registry. Am J Respir Crit Care Med 2016;193(1):68–77.
22. Silvestri GA, Bevill BT, Huang J, et al. An Evaluation of Diagnostic Yield From Bronchoscopy: The Impact of Clinical/Radiographic Factors, Procedure Type, and Degree of Suspicion for Cancer. Chest 2020;157(6):1656–64.
23. Tanner NT, Yarmus L, Chen A, et al. Standard Bronchoscopy With Fluoroscopy vs Thin Bronchoscopy and Radial Endobronchial Ultrasound for Biopsy of Pulmonary Lesions: A Multicenter, Prospective, Randomized Trial. Chest 2018;154(5):1035–43.
24. Asano F, Shinagawa N, Ishida T, et al. Virtual bronchoscopic navigation combined with ultrathin bronchoscopy. A randomized clinical trial. Am J Respir Crit Care Med 2013;188(3):327–33.
25. Eberhardt R, Anantham D, Ernst A, et al. Multimodality bronchoscopic diagnosis of peripheral lung lesions: a randomized controlled trial. Am J Respir Crit Care Med 2007;176(1):36–41.
26. Bhatt KM, Tandon YK, Graham R, et al. Electromagnetic Navigational Bronchoscopy versus CT-guided Percutaneous Sampling of Peripheral Indeterminate Pulmonary Nodules: A Cohort Study. Radiology 2018;286(3):1052–61.
27. DiBardino DM, Yarmus LB, Semaan RW. Transthoracic needle biopsy of the lung. J Thorac Dis 2015;7(Suppl 4):S304–16.
28. United States Food and Drug Administration. 501(k) Premarket notification - Ion Endoluminal System. 2019. Available at: https://www.accessdata.fda.gov/scripts/cdrh/cfdocs/cfpmn/pmn.cfm?ID=K192367. Accessed December 22, 2022.
29. United States Food and Drug Administration. 501(k) Premarket notification - Monarch Endoscopy Platform (Monarch Platform). 2018. Available at: https://www.accessdata.fda.gov/scripts/cdrh/cfdocs/cfpmn/pmn.cfm?ID=k173760. Accessed December 22, 2022.
30. Galloway KC, Chen Y, Templeton E, et al. Fiber Optic Shape Sensing for Soft Robotics. Soft Robot 2019;6(5):671–84.
31. Poeggel S, Tosi D, Duraibabu D, et al. Optical Fibre Pressure Sensors in Medical Applications. Sensors 2015;15(7):17115–48.
32. Rojas-Solano JR, Ugalde-Gamboa L, Machuzak M. Robotic Bronchoscopy for Diagnosis of Suspected Lung Cancer: A Feasibility Study. J Bronchology Interv Pulmonol 2018;25(3):168–75.
33. Chen AC, Pastis NJ, Mahajan AK, et al. Robotic Bronchoscopy for Peripheral Pulmonary Lesions: A Multicenter Pilot and Feasibility Study (BENEFIT). Chest 2021;159(2):845–52.
34. Chen AC, Gillespie CT. Robotic Endoscopic Airway Challenge: REACH Assessment. Ann Thorac Surg 2018;106(1):293–7.
35. Yarmus L, Akulian J, Wahidi M, et al. A Prospective Randomized Comparative Study of Three Guided Bronchoscopic Approaches for Investigating Pulmonary Nodules: The PRECISION-1 Study. Chest 2020;157(3):694–701.

36. Kapp CM, Akulian JA, Yu DH, et al. Cognitive Load in Electromagnetic Navigational and Robotic Bronchoscopy for Pulmonary Nodules. ATS Sch 2020; 2(1):97–107.
37. Fielding DIK, Bashirzadeh F, Son JH, et al. First Human Use of a New Robotic-Assisted Fiber Optic Sensing Navigation System for Small Peripheral Pulmonary Nodules. Respiration 2019;98(2): 142–50.
38. Benn BS, Romero AO, Lum M, et al. Robotic-Assisted Navigation Bronchoscopy as a Paradigm Shift in Peripheral Lung Access. Lung 2021;199(2):177–86.
39. Chaddha U, Kovacs SP, Manley C, et al. Robot-assisted bronchoscopy for pulmonary lesion diagnosis: results from the initial multicenter experience. BMC Pulm Med 2019;19(1):243.
40. Kalchiem-Dekel O, Connolly JG, Lin IH, et al. Shape-Sensing Robotic-Assisted Bronchoscopy in the Diagnosis of Pulmonary Parenchymal Lesions. Chest 2022;161(2):572–82.
41. Park CH, Han K, Hur J, et al. Comparative Effectiveness and Safety of Preoperative Lung Localization for Pulmonary Nodules: A Systematic Review and Meta-analysis. Chest 2017;151(2):316–28.
42. Lizza N, Eucher P, Haxhe JP, et al. Thoracoscopic resection of pulmonary nodules after computed tomographic-guided coil labeling. Ann Thorac Surg 2001;71(3):986–8.
43. Chen S, Zhou J, Zhang J, et al. Video-assisted thoracoscopic solitary pulmonary nodule resection after CT-guided hookwire localization: 43 cases report and literature review. Surg Endosc 2011;25(6):1723–9.
44. Doo KW, Yong HS, Kim HK, et al. Needlescopic resection of small and superficial pulmonary nodule after computed tomographic fluoroscopy-guided dual localization with radiotracer and hookwire. Ann Surg Oncol 2015;22(1):331–7.
45. Lin M-W, Tseng Y-H, Lee Y-F, et al. Computed tomography-guided patent blue vital dye localization of pulmonary nodules in uniportal thoracoscopy. J Thorac Cardiovasc Surg 2016;152(2):535–44.e2.
46. Yang Y-L, Li Z-Z, Huang W-C, et al. Electromagnetic navigation bronchoscopic localization versus percutaneous CT-guided localization for thoracoscopic resection of small pulmonary nodules. Thorac cancer 2021;12(4):468–74.
47. Yanagiya M, Kawahara T, Ueda K, et al. A meta-analysis of preoperative bronchoscopic marking for pulmonary nodules. Eur J Cardiothoracic Surg 2020;58(1):40–50.
48. Melfi FMA, Menconi GF, Mariani AM, et al. Early experience with robotic technology for thoracoscopic surgery. Eur J Cardiothoracic Surg 2002;21(5):864–8.
49. Tang A, Raja S, Bribriesco AC, et al. Robotic Approach Offers Similar Nodal Upstaging to Open Lobectomy for Clinical Stage I Non-small Cell Lung Cancer. Ann Thorac Surg 2020;110(2):424–33.
50. Kent M, Wang T, Whyte R, et al. Open, video-assisted thoracic surgery, and robotic lobectomy: review of a national database. Ann Thorac Surg 2014;97(1):234–6.
51. Cerfolio RJ, Bryant AS, Minnich DJ. Starting a robotic program in general thoracic surgery: why, how, and lessons learned. Ann Thorac Surg 2011;91(6):1727–9.
52. Giulianotti PC, Buchs NC, Caravaglios G, et al. Robot-assisted lung resection: outcomes and technical details. Interact Cardiovasc Thorac Surg 2010;11(4):388–92.
53. Kneuertz PJ, Singer E, D'Souza DM, et al. Hospital cost and clinical effectiveness of robotic-assisted versus video-assisted thoracoscopic and open lobectomy: A propensity score-weighted comparison. J Thorac Cardiovasc Surg 2019;157(5):2018–26.e2.
54. Deen SA, Wilson JL, Wilshire CL, et al. Defining the cost of care for lobectomy and segmentectomy: a comparison of open, video-assisted thoracoscopic, and robotic approaches. Ann Thorac Surg 2014; 97(3):1000–7.
55. Arnold BN, Thomas DC, Narayan R, et al. Robotic-Assisted Lobectomies in the National Cancer Database. J Am Coll Surg 2018;226(6):1052–62.e15.
56. Merritt RE, D'Souza DM, Abdel-Rasoul M, et al. Analysis of trends in perioperative outcomes in over 1000 robotic-assisted anatomic lung resections. J Robot Surg 2022. https://doi.org/10.1007/s11701-022-01436-3.
57. Onaitis MW, Furnary AP, Kosinski AS, et al. Equivalent Survival Between Lobectomy and Segmentectomy for Clinical Stage IA Lung Cancer. Ann Thorac Surg 2020;110(6):1882–91.
58. Suzuki K, Saji H, Aokage K, et al. Comparison of pulmonary segmentectomy and lobectomy: Safety results of a randomized trial. J Thorac Cardiovasc Surg 2019;158(3):895–907.
59. Kneuertz PJ, Singer E, D'Souza DM, et al. Postoperative complications decrease the cost-effectiveness of robotic-assisted lobectomy. Surgery 2019;165(2): 455–60.
60. Nguyen DM, Sarkaria IS, Song C, et al. Clinical and economic comparative effectiveness of robotic-assisted, video-assisted thoracoscopic, and open lobectomy. J Thorac Dis 2020;12(3):296–306.
61. Nasir BS, Bryant AS, Minnich DJ, et al. Performing robotic lobectomy and segmentectomy: cost, profitability, and outcomes. Ann Thorac Surg 2014;98(1): 203–9.
62. Singer E, Kneuertz PJ, D'Souza DM, et al. Understanding the financial cost of robotic lobectomy: calculating the value of innovation? Ann Cardiothorac Surg 2019;8(2):194–201.
63. Geraci TC, Ferrari-Light D, Kent A, et al. Technique, Outcomes With Navigational Bronchoscopy Using Indocyanine Green for Robotic Segmentectomy. Ann Thorac Surg 2019;108(2):363–9.

64. ROSS P, SKABLA P, SUTTER J, et al. Fast track nodule pathway: same day robotic diagnosis and resection. Chest 2021;160(4Supplement):A82.
65. Ross P, Skabla P, Sutter BJ, et al. Optimizing the resection pathway: can minimally invasive diagnosis and surgery (midas) guide patient selection? Chest 2022;162(4 Supplement):A1615.
66. Kern KA. Medicolegal analysis of the delayed diagnosis of cancer in 338 cases in the United States. Arch Surg 1994;129(4):394–7.
67. Institute of Medicine (US) Committee on Quality of Health Care in America. Crossing the Quality Chasm: A New Health System for the 21st Century. Washington (DC): National Academies Press (US); 2001. doi:10.17226/10027.
68. Asch SM, Kerr EA, Hamilton EG, et al. McGlynn eds Quality of care for oncologic conditions and HIV: a review of the literature and quality indicators. Santa Monica, CA: RAND Corporation; 2000.
69. Field J, deKoning H, Oudkerk M, et al. Implementation of lung cancer screening in Europe: Challenges and potential solutions: Summary of a multidisciplinary roundtable discussion. ESMO Open 2019;4:e000577.
70. (NICE) NIFH and CE. National Collaborating Centre for Cancer. Lung Cancer. The Diagnosis and Treatment of Lung Cancer. 2011th ed. London, Cardiff (UK);. 2011.
71. Jacobsen MM, Silverstein SC, Quinn M, et al. Timeliness of access to lung cancer diagnosis and treatment: A scoping literature review. Lung Cancer 2017;112:156–64.
72. Linford G, Egan R, Coderre-Ball A, et al. Patient and physician perceptions of lung cancer care in a multidisciplinary clinic model. Curr Oncol 2020;27(1):e9–19.
73. Stone CJL, Vaid HM, Selvam R, et al. Multidisciplinary Clinics in Lung Cancer Care: A Systematic Review. Clin Lung Cancer 2018;19(4):323–30.e3.

# Bronchoscopic Lung Volume Reduction
## A Clinical Review

Shourjo Chakravorty, MD[a], Mahwish Bari, BS[b],
Duy Kevin Duong, MD, DAABIP[c], Priya P. Patel, MD, DAABIP[c],
Amit K. Mahajan, MD, FCCP, DAABIP[d,*]

**KEYWORDS**

• Bronchoscopic lung volume reduction • Endobronchial valves • Emphysema

**KEY POINTS**

- Endobronchial valves (EBVs) for bronchoscopic lung volume reduction (BLVR) are an advancing "guideline treatment" in the treatment of advanced emphysema. Placement of small, one-way valves into segmental or subsegmental airways can induce lobar atelectasis for portions of diseased lung.
- Appropriate patient selection is essential for procedural success using EBV.
- Patient functionality is significantly improved using BLVR by both objective and subjective measurements.

## INTRODUCTION

Pulmonary emphysema is a form of chronic obstructive pulmonary disease (COPD), which is typically related to cigarette smoking.[1] The pathophysiology of the disease process involves abnormal and irreversible enlargement of the air sacs distal to the terminal bronchioles.[2] As the thin walls of the alveolar air sacs are destroyed over time, pulmonary elasticity is lost, thus impairing normal airflow mechanics. As elasticity is lost, patients lose the ability to effectively move air out, eventually leading to air trapping and hyperinflation.[3] Hyperinflation of the lungs results in flattening of the diaphragm. Flattening of the diaphragm makes it difficult to generate adequate negative pressure to effectively inspire. Manifestations of emphysema are broad, as some patients are asymptomatic when disease is mild, whereas some have significant dyspnea at rest, productive cough, chest tightness, wheezing, and weakness.[3]

Despite advances in primary and secondary prevention, emphysema remains a major cause of morbidity and mortality globally. Lung volume reduction surgery (LVRS) is an invasive intervention to reduce hyperinflation by resecting hyperinflated portions of the lung. Many patients with emphysema are unable to tolerate the morbidity and complication profile of LVRS.[4] One major advancement in treatment for emphysema is the use of endobronchial valves (EBV). EBVs are small, one-way valves that are placed in segmental or subsegmental airways to induce lobar atelectasis and improve lung function, dyspnea, and quality of life[5] (**Fig. 1**).

## PATHOPHYSIOLOGY OF EMPHYSEMA

In healthy lungs, this intrinsic quality of elastic recoil allows for easy exhalation. As the alveolar walls are damaged and destroyed, elastic recoil is lost. In emphysema, decreased elastic recoil leads to increased airway resistance and increased

[a] Department of Medicine, Inova Fairfax Medical Center, Falls Church, VA, USA; [b] Lung/Interventional Pulmonology, Inova Schar Cancer Institute, Falls Church, VA, USA; [c] Department of Interventional Pulmonology, Inova Schar Cancer Institute, Inova Fairfax Hospital, Falls Church, VA, USA; [d] Interventional Pulmonology, Department of Surgery, Inova Schar Cancer Institute, Inova Fairfax Hospital, Falls Church, VA, USA
* Corresponding author. 8081 Innovation Park Drive, Fairfax, VA 22031.
*E-mail address:* amit.mahajan@inova.org

Thorac Surg Clin 33 (2023) 245–250
https://doi.org/10.1016/j.thorsurg.2023.04.014

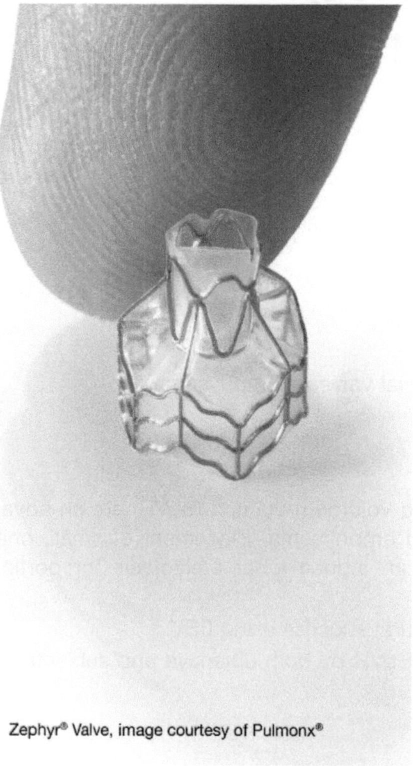


**Fig. 1.** One-way Zephyr (Pulmonx Corp) endobronchial valve. (*Courtesy of* Pulmonx Corp, Redwood, CA.)

compliance, which result in inefficient airflow and obstructive physiology. Over time, air trapping and lung hyperinflation contribute to dyspnea, exercise intolerance, muscular weakness, and increase morbidity. COPD-related dyspnea is related to numerous, complex, and overlapping mechanisms, which include airway obstruction with expiratory flow limitations, both static and dynamic hyperinflation, increased respiratory muscle load, changes in respiratory drive, peripheral muscle weakness, and pulmonary vascular changes.[6] In addition, due to increased airway resistance, there is early closure of the small airways during expiration, which contributes to air-trapping and increased residual volume (RV).[7] Chronic airflow limitation imposes a load on respiratory muscles, flattening the diaphragm and reducing its ability to generate tension.[8] Emphysema and hyperinflation also lead to changes in chest wall geometry and diaphragm position which also contributes to respiratory muscle dysfunction.[8] Diaphragmatic weakness and immobility have been shown to be correlated with dyspnea as chest wall muscles are recruited to generate negative intrathoracic pressure.[9] Over time, air trapping and lung hyperinflation contribute to dyspnea, exercise intolerance, muscular weakness, and increase morbidity. This is often accompanied by severe dyspnea, which over time can lead to a spiral of avoiding physical activity intolerance, physical deconditioning, reduced quality of life, and subsequent increase in early development of cardiovascular disease.[10]

## ENDOBRONCHIAL VALVES

EBV placement for emphysema was initially developed in the early 2000s as a minimally invasive alternative to LVRS.[11] One-way valves are implanted in airways to allow exhaled air to flow easily through a valve and out of the lobe while preventing air from entering the treated lobe.[12] This results in lobe atelectasis in the absence of ventilation from the ipsilateral, untreated lobe, known as collateral ventilation.[13] By inducing lobar atelectasis for portions of diseased lung, hyperinflation is reduced resulting in improved diaphragmatic curvature and excursion.[14] This improvement in diaphragmatic function results in improved functionality and pulmonary function.[5]

EBVs present as an advancing "guideline treatment" for advanced emphysema. This recommendation stemmed from 2 decades of randomized controlled trials investigating safety and efficacy, selection criteria, and procedural and postprocedure

**Box 1**
**General inclusion criteria for bronchoscopic lung volume reduction**

- History of emphysema
- Body mass index (BMI) less than 35 kg/m$^2$
- Stable with less than or equal to 20 mg of prednisone daily
- Radiographic evidence of emphysema on high-resolution computed tomography scan
- Forced expiratory volume in 1 second (FEV1, % predicted) less than or equal to 45% predicted or greater than or equal to 15% predicted
- Total lung capacity greater than or equal to 100% predicted post-bronchodilator
- Residual volume greater than or equal to 175% predicted post-bronchodilator
- Six-minute walk distance greater than or equal to 100 m and less than 500 m
- Nonsmoking for 4 months before initial interview and throughout evaluation for the procedure
- Able to tolerate anesthesia safely
- The lobe targeted for treatment must have little to no collateral ventilation

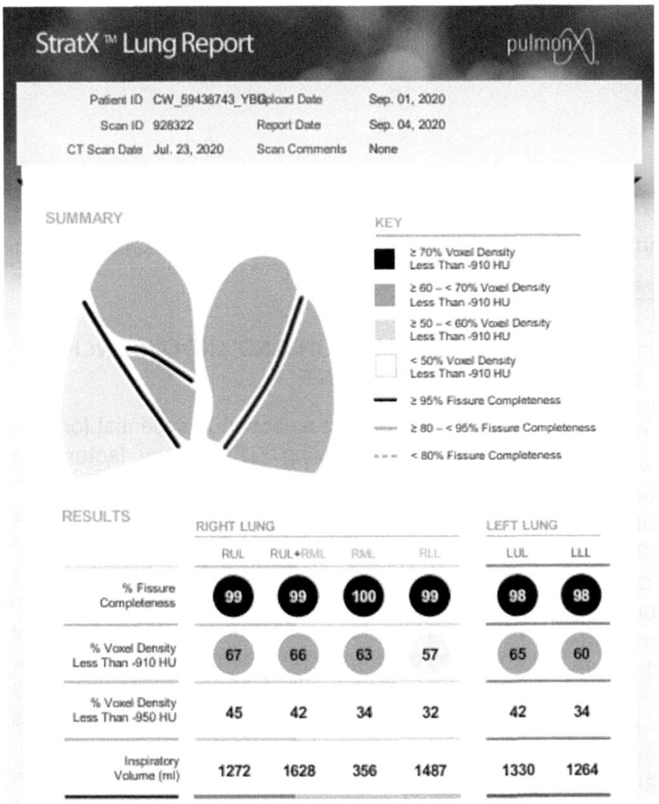


**Fig. 2.** Analysis of lung destruction, volumes, and fissure integrity. (*Courtesy of* Pulmonx Corp, Redwood, CA.)

management. The Endobronchial Valve for Emphysema Palliation Trial (VENT) was the principle study to examine symptom improvement, safety, and efficacy of Zephyr EBVs treatment of emphysema.[15] Designed in parallel to the LVRS study National Emphysema Treatment Trial (NETT), 270 VENT study patients were randomized 2:1 to either the EBV implantation group or the optimal medical management program as defined by the 2001 National Institutes of Health/World Health Organization Global Initiative for Chronic Obstructive Lung Disease (GOLD) guidelines group[16] or the control group receiving GOLD-guided medical management only.[16] Forced expiratory volume in 1 second (FEV1) averaged an increase of 4.3% in the EBV treatment group compared with a 2.5% decrease in FEV1 in the control group resulting in mean arm difference of 6.8% ($P = .005$) at the 6-month evaluation mark. Complication rates (including COPD exacerbation, pneumonia, hemoptysis, and pneumothorax) at the 1-year mark was 10.3% in the treatment group as compared with 4.6% in the control ($P = .17$).[17] The VENT trial showed improved outcomes in FEV1 and exercise tolerance in patients with advanced emphysema along with acceptable postprocedure exacerbations of COPD and adverse events.[15]

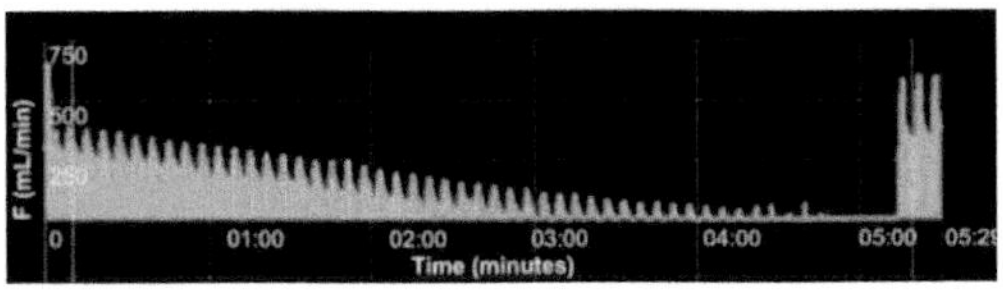


**Fig. 3.** Chartis analysis of intraoperative airflow to determine the presence of collateral ventilation. Reducing flow, seen below, is representative of negative collateral ventilation. (*Courtesy of* Pulmonx Corp, Redwood, CA.)

The Spiration Valve System (SVS) is an umbrella shaped one-way valve that limits airflow to distal, emphysema-affected areas of lung.[18] Spiration valve implementation in patients with severe heterogeneous emphysema was the focus of the EMPROVE trial, Improving Lung Function in Severe Heterogeneous Emphysema with the SVS.[19] This represented the largest multicenter valve study to use high-resolution computer tomography (HRCT) analysis of fissure integrity for patient selection for lobular treatment.[18] One-hundred and seventy-two EMPROVE study patients were randomized 2:1 to either the SVS and medical management treatment group or the medical management control group. As compared with previous SVS trials using bilateral partial occlusion which did not yield significant

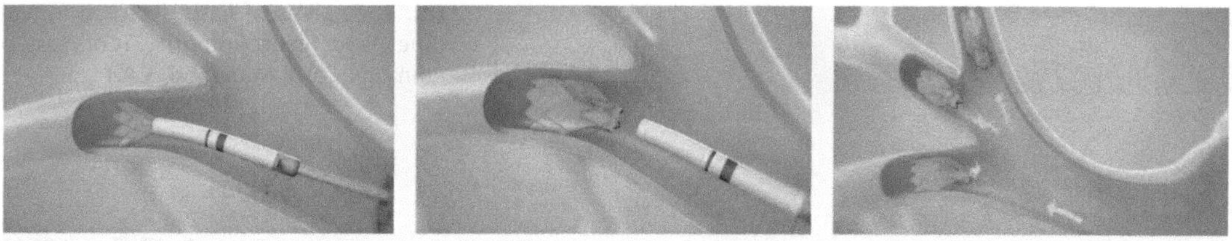


**Fig. 4.** Deployment catheters used to place endobronchial valves for BLVR. (*Courtesy of* Pulmonx Corp, Redwood, CA.)

improvements, the EMPROVE trial resulted in significant improvements including reductions in total lung volume (TLV), hyperinflation, and dyspnea. The FEV1 in the SVS group increased by 0.099 L on average from baseline as compared with the −0.002 L difference from the control treatment group. Of note, the EMPROVE trial's usage of quantitative HRCT analysis for fissure integrity ≥90% as an inclusionary factor in patient selection demonstrated improvements in FEV1, hyperinflation, TLV, dyspnea, and quality of life (QoL) measures in comparison to the control medical treatment group alone.[20]

Zephyr EBV valves became approved by the Food and Drug Administration in 2018 as a result of significant data collection within the LIBERATE (Lung Function Improvement after Bronchoscopic Lung Volume Reduction With Pulmonx Endobronchial Valves Used in Treatment of Emphysema) trial.[18] LIBERATE was the first multicenter randomized control trial to investigate the safety and effectiveness of the Zephyr EBVs in patient group with little or no collateral ventilation between the treated and the ipsilateral lobe over 12 months.[19] Hundred and ninety study subjects were randomized 2:1 to either EBV and standard medical management group or the control arm of standard medical management. Considering greater than or equal to 15% increase over baseline of post-bronchodilator FEV, 47.7% patients receiving EBV met the benchmark as compared with 16.8% control group patients, with a between group difference of 31.0. Of note, of the EBV treatment group 79.1% study patients reached minimally clinically important difference for total lung volume reduction at the 45-day mark and 84.2% patients at the 12-month mark. The absence of collateral ventilation was confirmed before valve implantation using the Chartis system, which detects airflow in a target lobe. There was an average 1.14 L reduction in total target lobe volume measured by HRCT in the EBV treatment group, resulting in a mean RV reduction of 0.5 L (decreased 10.38% from baseline).[19] The LIBERATE trial identified the most common major short-term side effect following EBV implantation to be pneumothorax.[19]

## PATIENT SELECTION AND ENDOBRONCHIAL VALVE PLACEMENT

Appropriate patient selection is essential for procedural success using EBVs. Many factors are included in determining if a patient is an acceptable candidate for bronchoscopic lung volume reduction (BLVR). General inclusion criteria are shown in **Box 1**. Patients with a heterogenous pattern of emphysema based on the comparison of ipsilateral lobar destruction tend to have improved outcomes compared with those with homogenous disease.[19] If these basic inclusion criteria are met for BLVR therapy, further analysis is obtained using a high-resolution computed tomography scan to assess lobar volume, degree of destruction from emphysema, and fissure completeness (**Figs. 2** and **3**). Fissure completeness is an indicator of collateral ventilation between ipsilateral lobes. Although multiple physiologic components are considered for treatment, fissure completeness is among the most important, as was demonstrated in the LIBERATE trial. Intraprocedural confirmation that no collateral ventilation is present can be achieved using airflow assessment platforms, such as the Chartis system (see **Fig. 2**). In the presence of complete fissures, the placement of EBVs can result in complete target lobe atelectasis. Reduction in hyperinflation

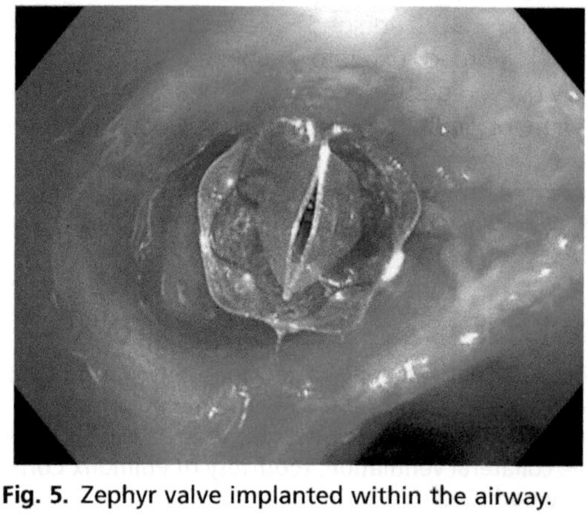

**Fig. 5.** Zephyr valve implanted within the airway.

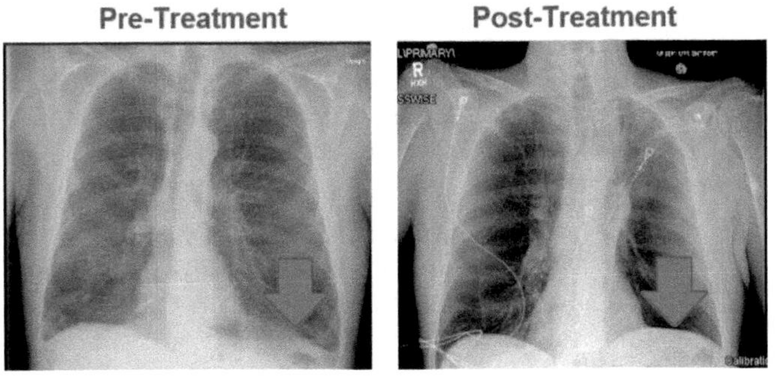


**Fig. 6.** Post-BLVR chest x-ray. Pre-BLVR on right. Post-BLVR on left. Improvement in left diaphragmatic curvature following valve placement (arrow).

from target lobe atelectasis improves hemidiaphragm curvature, increases diaphragmatic excursion, and reduces work of breathing.

Patients are traditionally intubated and sedated for EBV placement. Various ventilation techniques can be used to ensure patient safety and minimize the risk of complications following the procedure, namely pneumothorax. The procedure can be performed in either a bronchoscopy suite or operating room depending on the proceduralist level of comfort.

The placement of EBVs requires advanced bronchoscopy skills, familiarity with airway measurement equipment, and an understanding of airway anatomy. Although two valve devices are currently available for use, Zephyr and Spiration require accurate measurements of airway depth and diameter to assign appropriate valve size. Various catheters and airway sizing devices are available, with different mechanisms of use. After the valve size has been chosen for a specific airway, valves are deployed into the airway for occlusion (**Fig. 4**). The appropriate number of valves is placed to occlude all segmental or subsegmental airway of the target lobe (**Fig. 5**). A complete occlusion of the target lobe will result in lobar atelectasis if the procedure is performed properly, resulting in improved diaphragmatic curvature (**Fig. 6**).

Major complications in the immediate postprocedure setting include pneumothorax and respiratory failure. Although appropriate patient selection should minimize the incidence of acute respiratory failure following the procedure, pneumothorax can be seen in as many as 26% of patients undergoing EBV therapy. According to the LIBERATE trial, most of pneumothoraces occur in the first 72 hours following treatment. As a result, it is highly encouraged for physicians to be comfortable with chest tube placement. In addition, appropriate knowledge of chest tube management in the setting of a persistent air leaks is necessary to ensure that the best patient outcomes are achieved. Exacerbation of underlying COPD can occur but is typically seen on postoperative day 1 or 2.

## SUMMARY

Severe emphysema is a source of significant morbidity and mortality. Millions of people around the world suffer from emphysema and must live with the debilitating consequences of the disease. The advent of BLVR has offered a minimally invasive and effective option capable of reducing air-trapping and improving diaphragmatic function. The placement of EBVs emulates the effects of LVRS, without the associated morbidity and potential mortality. As a result, patient functionality is significantly improved using BLVR by both objective and subjective measurements. As the procedure continues to gain popularity, the phenotype of patients who may benefit from BLVR will become more apparent. With additional research and clinical utilization, many more individuals will experience the benefits of this revolutionary treatment.

## CLINICS CARE POINTS

- Bronchoscopic lung volume reduction (BLVR) is an effective treatment of patients with emphysema.
- A growing body of evidence exists supporting the use of BLVR.

## DISCLOSURE

Dr A.K. Mahajan is an educational consultant for Pulmonx Corporation. All other authors have no disclosures.

## REFERENCES

1. Hogg JC, Timens W. The pathology of chronic obstructive pulmonary disease. Annu Rev Pathol 2009;4:435–59.
2. Pahal P, Avula A, Sharma S. Emphysema. In: StatPearls. Treasure Island (FL): StatPearls Publishing; 2022.

3. Barnes PJ, Burney PG, Silverman EK, et al. Chronic obstructive pulmonary disease. Nat Rev Dis Primers 2015;1:15076.
4. Shah PL, Herth FJ, van Geffen WH, et al. Lung volume reduction for emphysema. Lancet Respir Med 2017;5(2):147–56 [Erratum in: Lancet Respir Med. 2016;4(11):e55].
5. Slebos DJ, Shah PL, Herth FJ, et al. Endobronchial Valves for Endoscopic Lung Volume Reduction: Best Practice Recommendations from Expert Panel on Endoscopic Lung Volume Reduction. Respiration 2017;93(2):138–50.
6. Petrovic M, Reiter M, Zipko H, et al. Effects of inspiratory muscle training on dynamic hyperinflation in patients with COPD. Int J Chron Obstruct Pulmon Dis 2012;7:797–805.
7. Burgel PR. The role of small airways in obstructive airway diseases. Eur Respir Rev 2011;20(119): 23–33 [Erratum in: Eur Respir Rev. 2011;20(120): 123. Dosage error in article text. Erratum in: Eur Respir Rev. 2011;20(120):124].
8. Santana PV, Albuquerque ALP. Respiratory muscles in COPD: be aware of the diaphragm. J Bras Pneumol 2018;44(1):1–2.
9. Dubé BP, Dres M. Diaphragm Dysfunction: Diagnostic Approaches and Management Strategies. J Clin Med 2016;5(12):113.
10. Wüst RC, Degens H. Factors contributing to muscle wasting and dysfunction in COPD patients. Int J Chron Obstruct Pulmon Dis 2007;2(3):289–300.
11. Hartman JE, Vanfleteren LEGW, van Rikxoort EM, et al. Endobronchial valves for severe emphysema. Eur Respir Rev 2019;28(152):180121.
12. Wang R, Paul S, Truong V, et al. Bronchoscopic interventions for emphysema: Current status. Lung India 2020;37(6):518–29.
13. Klooster K, Slebos DJ. Endobronchial Valves for the Treatment of Advanced Emphysema. Chest 2021; 159(5):1833–42.
14. Dransfield MT, Garner JL, Bhatt SP, et al, LIBERATE Study Group. Effect of Zephyr Endobronchial Valves on Dyspnea, Activity Levels, and Quality of Life at One Year. Results from a Randomized Clinical Trial. Ann Am Thorac Soc 2020;17(7):829–38.
15. Strange C, Herth FJ, Kovitz KL, et al. Design of the Endobronchial Valve for Emphysema Palliation Trial (VENT): a non-surgical method of lung volume reduction. BMC Pulm Med 2007;7:10. https://doi.org/10.1186/1471-2466-7-10.
16. Pauwels RA, Buist AS, Calverley PM, et al, GOLD Scientific Committee. Global strategy for the diagnosis, management, and prevention of chronic obstructive pulmonary disease. NHLBI/WHO Global Initiative for Chronic Obstructive Lung Disease (GOLD) Workshop summary. Am J Respir Crit Care Med 2001;163(5):1256–76.
17. Sciurba FC, Ernst A, Herth FJ, et al. A Randomized Study of Endobronchial Valves for Advanced Emphysema. N Engl J Med 2010;363(13):1233–44. https://doi.org/10.1056/nejmoa0900928.
18. Nada KM, Nishi S. Endoscopic Lung Volume Reduction: Review of the EMPROVE and LIBERATE trials. Mayo Clin Proc Innov Qual Outcomes 2020;5(1): 177–86.
19. Criner GJ, Sue R, Wright S, et al, LIBERATE Study Group. A Multicenter Randomized Controlled Trial of Zephyr Endobronchial Valve Treatment in Heterogeneous Emphysema (LIBERATE). Am J Respir Crit Care Med 2018;198(9):1151–64.
20. Criner GJ, Delage A, Voelker K, et al. Improving Lung Function in Severe Heterogenous Emphysema with the Spiration Valve System (EMPROVE). A Multicenter, Open-Label Randomized Controlled Clinical Trial. Am J Respir Crit Care Med 2019; 200(11):1354–62.

# Advanced Endoscopy for Thoracic Surgeons

Kathleen M.I. Fuentes, MD[a], Kenneth P. Seastedt, MD[b], Biniam Kidane, MD[c], Elliot L. Servais, MD[d,*]

**KEYWORDS**

• Endoscopy • Peroral endoscopic myotomy • Endoluminal vacuum therapy • Endoscopic stenting • Endoscopic clip • Anastomotic leak • Esophageal perforation

**KEY POINTS**

- Several endoscopic techniques have been demonstrated to be noninferior to traditional foregut surgical options, such as peroral endoscopic myotomy for achalasia.
- Other evolving endoscopic therapies include endoscopic stenting, endoluminal vacuum therapy, endoscopic internal drainage, and endoscopic suturing/clipping.
- Endoscopic options for management are evolving, and the thoracic surgeon should continue to incorporate these techniques as well as drive future endoscopic innovations.

**Video content accompanies this article at http://www.thoracic.theclinics.com.**

## BACKGROUND

Endoscopic evaluation in medicine dates back at least to the time of Hippocrates and is now a necessary armament in the surgeon's toolkit. Classically, the endoscope was used to localize lesions for diagnosis and operative planning; however, endoscopic interventions and endoluminal surgical techniques are rapidly expanding, and the thoracic surgeon must remain aware of these advances and at the forefront of these procedures.[1] Endoscopic mucosal/submucosal dissection (EMR/ESD) for treating early-stage esophageal cancer is now the standard of care, with excellent reviews available elsewhere.[2] Relevant advances discussed in this article include endoscopic treatments for diseases such as achalasia, Zenker diverticula, esophageal diverticula, gastric outlet obstruction/gastroparesis, and esophageal perforations and leaks.

## ESOPHAGEAL ANATOMY

The esophagus connects the pharynx to the stomach, serving to transport swallowed food, and is approximately 25 cm long, starting at the cricoid and ending at the gastric cardia. The esophagus has several layers: epithelium, basement membrane, lamina propria, muscularis mucosa, submucosa, muscularis propria, and adventitia. Many endoscopic techniques exploit the loose submucosal connective tissue layer between the mucosa and the muscular layer. There are natural constrictions of the esophagus, the narrowest being at the upper esophageal sphincter, with the other constrictions being from the arch of the aorta and at the diaphragmatic hiatus. The most common esophageal diverticula, Zenker diverticula, is a false pulsion diverticulum that occurs through a weakness in Killian triangle at the inferior

[a] Department of General Surgery, Lahey Hospital and Medical Center, 41 Mall Road, Burlington, MA 01805, USA; [b] Department of Surgery, Beth Israel Deaconess Medical Center, Harvard Medical School, 330 Brookline Avenue, Boston, MA 02215, USA; [c] Department of Surgery, University of Manitoba, Room GE-611, 820 Sherbook Street, Winnipeg, Manitoba R3A 1R9, Canada; [d] Division of Thoracic Surgery, Lahey Hospital and Medical Center, 41 Mall Road, Burlington, MA 01805, USA
* Corresponding author.
*E-mail address:* elliot.servais@lahey.org

Thorac Surg Clin 33 (2023) 251–263
https://doi.org/10.1016/j.thorsurg.2023.04.015

pharyngeal constrictor and cricopharyngeus muscles of the hypopharynx. Traction diverticula are usually caused by mediastinal inflammation and occur midesophagus, with epiphrenic diverticula being false pulsion diverticula near the esophageal hiatus. The lower esophageal sphincter (LES) is a poorly defined anatomic zone under neurohormonal control with multiple components contributing to adequate esophageal closure: esophageal muscle and sling fibers of the gastric cardia, the phrenoesophageal ligament, and the diaphragmatic crura. The esophagus does not have a dedicated arterial supply; however, it comes from surrounding vessels off the aorta, with a rich venous drainage plexus in the adventitia and submucosa that drains to the azygous, hemiazygous, and gastric veins. Lymph drainage goes to nodes surrounding the esophagus, within the mediastinum, and the lesser curve of the stomach. Although often variable, in general, lymph flow at the cervical esophagus goes to deep cervical nodes, the thoracic esophagus above the carina drains upward to mediastinal nodes, and lymph drainage inferior to the carina drains caudally to the abdomen.[3]

## DIAGNOSIS

Esophageal pathologic condition can encompass a variety of clinical presentations, including dysphagia, chest pain, heartburn, regurgitation, weight loss, and dyspnea, among others. Several tools can aid in diagnosing esophageal pathologic condition, including barium or water-soluble swallow studies, endoscopy, computed tomography (CT), esophageal manometry, impedance testing, pH testing, as well as various studies evaluating the stomach, such as gastric-emptying studies. One of the significant endoscopic advances for the treatment of thoracic disease is for dysphagia, and causes of esophageal dysphagia include structural issues, such as stricture, extrinsic compression, and esophageal cancer, all of which can be identified on upper endoscopy. If swallow studies/CT/endoscopy do not identify a cause of dysphagia, manometry can help identify a cause. These can be classified into motility disorders or disorders of incomplete LES relaxation, such as achalasia and esophagogastric junction outflow obstruction (achalasia in evolution). Achalasia subcategories based on high-resolution manometry include type I (aperistalsis), type II (panesophageal pressurization), and type III (spastic).[4] Treatment options fall into 2 main categories: surgical and nonsurgical. Nonsurgical treatment options include pneumatic dilation (PD) and medications, such as nitroglycerin, calcium channel blockers, nitrates, and Botox injections.[5] Surgical options include esophagomyotomy with partial fundoplication, which can be performed laparoscopically or with robotic assistance, and, more recently, peroral endoscopic myotomy (POEM).

## PERORAL ENDOSCOPIC MYOTOMY

As initially described in humans by Inoue and colleagues,[6] POEM has become an alternative for treating achalasia. POEM uses endoscopy to perform the equivalent of a surgical myotomy in a less-invasive manner. Both modalities do not offer curative treatment but equally aim to reduce LES pressure, reduce esophageal spasm, and improve symptoms of dysphagia.

When comparing endoscopic treatment options, such as PD and POEM, POEM is a more durable intervention, given that PD, by its nature, requires repeat dilations. Eckardt scores are considered a standard by which to compare treatment modalities for achalasia.[7] A systematic review comparing PD with POEM showed that short-term outcomes based on self-reported reflux and dysphagia by Eckardt score favor POEM over PD.[8]

Several trials have compared long-term outcomes of POEM versus laparoscopic Heller myotomy with partial fundoplication (LHM-PF). In a recent systematic review, improvement of dysphagia was reported in 93.2% of patients who underwent POEM and 87.7% for those who underwent LHM-PF.[9] In one randomized controlled trial comparing POEM with LHM-PF at a single center, equivalent control of clinical symptoms at follow-up at 1, 6, and 12 months was found.[10] The noninferiority of POEM to LHM-PF was also corroborated in a larger randomized controlled trial across several centers. An Eckardt symptom score of 3 or less was considered a clinical success, and this trial demonstrated that POEM had 82.4% clinical success at 2 years and LHM-PF had 80.6% (not statistically significant).[11] Overall, these results demonstrate the noninferiority of POEM to LHM-PF in treating dysphagia symptoms.

POEM does not involve a concurrent antireflux procedure, and the decreased LES tone allows for more retrograde reflux of stomach contents. In the aforementioned single-center randomized controlled trial, reflux symptoms were significantly higher in the POEM group (64.6% vs 11.1%).[10] This was also reflected in a systematic review comparing POEM with LHM-PF, showing significantly more gastroesophageal reflux disease (GERD) symptoms by erosive esophagitis, pH monitoring, and patient-reported symptoms.[9] In the larger randomized controlled trial, 44% of patients who underwent POEM had reflux esophagitis by 24 months, compared with 29% in the LHM-PF group.[11] The long-term consequences of increased reflux after POEM have not been established. Potential increased reflux is an important consideration for patients to be aware of when considering this procedure versus LHM-PF.

Rate of reintervention is another important outcome metric when comparing achalasia treatments. PD generally requires repeat interventions, as the procedure itself only temporarily relieves the increased LES tone, demonstrated across several studies.[8] In contrast, reintervention rates for treatment failures between POEM and LHM-PF are similar.[11]

In 2 randomized controlled trials, procedure time and anesthesia time were significantly shorter in patients undergoing POEM over LHM-PF. However, there was no significant difference in hospital length of stay in either study.[10,11] Surprisingly, in one systematic review, hospital length of stay was greater in patients undergoing POEM (1.03 days longer; $P = .04$).[9] This could be explained by selection bias for POEM over LHM-PF, given that POEM may have been offered to patients who were less-ideal candidates for a more-invasive procedure. In addition, another contributor to prolonged length of stay with POEM is likely provider inexperience and hesitation to discharge given the novelty of POEM, which, on more experience with POEM, is reflected in the randomized controlled trial showing an equivalent length of stay as providers gain more experience with the procedure, its complications, and postprocedural management.

Despite drawbacks related to gastroesophageal reflux, POEM has similar or decreased rates of adverse events to other available procedural achalasia treatment options. Large-scale evaluation of adverse events in POEM shows a rate of 7.5% to 9.4%.[12,13] In comparison to LHM-PF, POEM has fewer serious adverse events.[10,11] Large-scale studies have similar adverse event rates, with one study including 3135 patients and an adverse event rate of 8.23%. Complications included mucosal barrier failure, delayed bleeding, pleural effusion, pneumothorax, and others (inflammation, stroke, coma).[14]

Therefore, POEM offers a safe and effective treatment for patients with esophageal outlet diseases, which is at worse noninferior to traditional surgical intervention. Careful consideration must be given to a patient's overall health, ability to tolerate prolonged anesthesia, and long-term risks/benefits as outlined above. PD is a good option for patients who cannot tolerate general anesthesia but requires repeat dilations. Both LHM-PF and POEM offer longer-term symptom relief, but one must weigh the risks of intra-abdominal operation versus an increase in gastroesophageal reflux in considering these interventions.

## *Peroral Endoscopic Myotomy Technique*

At the authors' institution, they recommend the following instrumentation and settings:

- 25-gauge articulator injection needle
- Olympus cap attachment for gastroscope
- Endo Cut Q effect 3, cut duration 1, cut interval 1(Erbe USA Inc, Marietta, GA, USA)
- Spray coagulation effect 2, Watts 40
- HybridKnife I-type I-jet, Erbe Jet effect 25, suction −1.5 (Erbe USA Inc)
- Pump cartridge for Erbe Jet 2 (Erbe USA Inc)

See Video 1 for the authors' POEM technique demonstration. To begin, they perform an upper endoscopy and evaluate the esophagus and stomach. It is important to ensure no evidence of esophageal malignancy that may lead to pseudoachalasia. In addition, they ensure the integrity of the esophageal and gastric mucosa without significant esophagitis, which could increase the risk of mucosal perforation. The authors then retract the endoscope approximately 15 cm from the LES and inject methylene blue into submucosal space, taking care to inject sufficient methylene blue (approximately 6–7 mL) to adequately lift the submucosa off of the muscle layers to facilitate entering and forming the tunnel to advance the endoscope (**Fig. 1**). Using the hybrid knife, they then cut into the mucosa for the initial mucosotomy (**Fig. 2**). The authors then inject additional methylene blue after entering the mucosotomy to create additional space to aid in the advancement of the scope. Advancing into this plane, the underlying muscle layer is used to verify the correct plane and the blue-tinted submucosal layer (**Fig. 3**).

The authors then orient the gastroscope, so the circular muscle is oriented at the 6 o'clock position with the mucosa at 12 o'clock. They continue to inject methylene blue to raise the mucosa off the muscular layer while using the hybrid knife on the coagulation setting to divide the submucosa as the gastroscope is advanced into the tunnel. Several small vessels may be encountered upon advancing, which can be coagulated using the hybrid knife. Large vessels should not be coagulated directly to avoid bleeding into the surgical field but should be dissected on either side with coagulation to create space for a coagulation

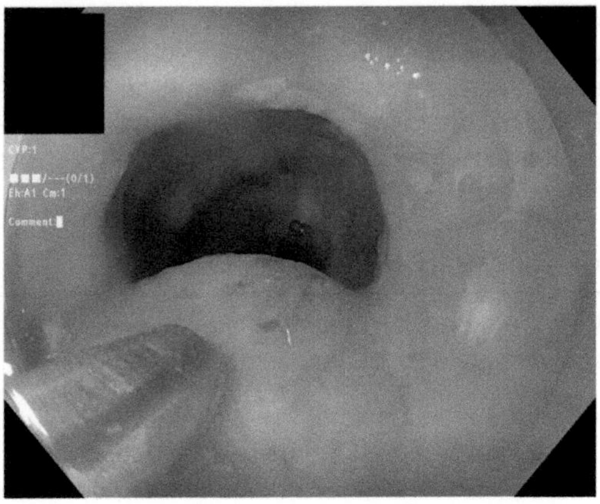

**Fig. 1.** Submucosal methylene blue injection.

grasper. To safely divide these vessels, the authors use a coagulation grasper to first cauterize, and the vessel can then be cut with the hybrid knife (**Fig. 4**).

On approach to the LES, the fibers of the muscle change direction, and the authors stain the mucosa with methylene blue in this area (**Fig. 5**). They then exit the tunnel, enter the true lumen of the esophagus and enter the stomach, and visualize the methylene blue near the cardia of the stomach by retroflexion to confirm the location below the LES and sufficient distal extent of submucosal tunneling. They then reenter the submucosal plane and begin the myotomy 2 to 3 cm distal from the mucosotomy, as these locations should not overlap. The authors divide the circular muscles while attempting to maintain the longitudinal muscles (**Fig. 6**). This can be difficult to maintain, as the musculature splays as they are divided. A full-thickness myotomy is often encountered and is not a problem so long as the mucosotomy is completely closed at the end of the procedure.

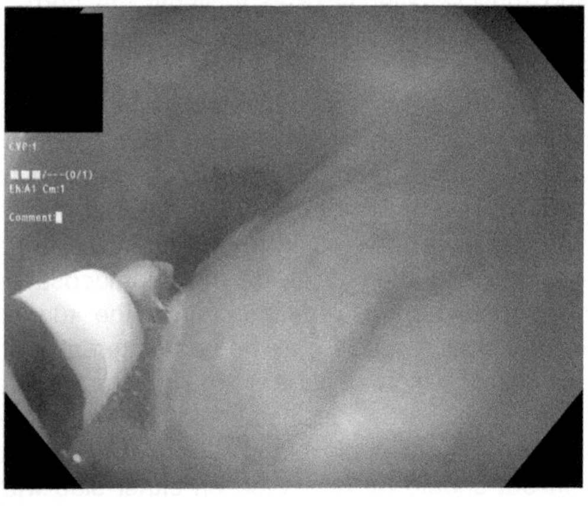

**Fig. 2.** POEM mucosotomy.

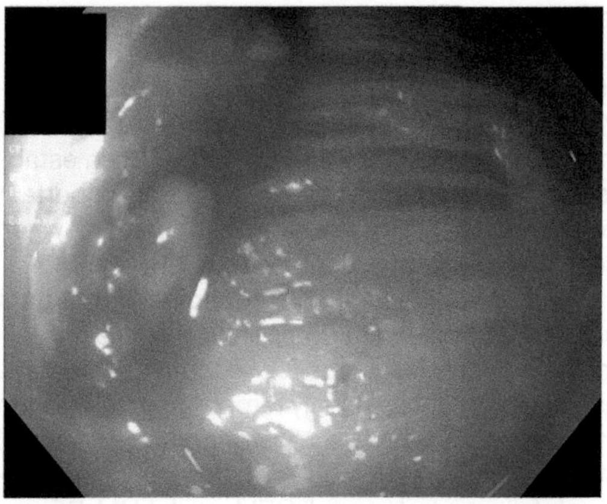

**Fig. 3.** Muscle layer visualization confirming proper submucosal plane.

They continue the myotomy with care to not cause thermal injury to the mucosa down to the gastric cardia. On completion, the scope is removed from the submucosal tunnel and advanced in the true lumen through the LES to confirm adequate and complete myotomy by sensing the decrease in tone at the LES and the ease with which the gastroscope can enter the stomach. Finally, the authors use endoscopic clips to close the mucosotomy (**Fig. 7**).[15] Although not included in the video, sometimes pneumoperitoneum may result secondary to a full-thickness myotomy. Uncommonly, this can cause an increase in end-tidal $CO_2$ or peak inspiratory pressures and may require decompression of the abdomen with a Veress needle.

## *Peroral Endoscopic Myotomy Variations*

Several other endoscopic interventions use the principles of the POEM technique to treat a variety

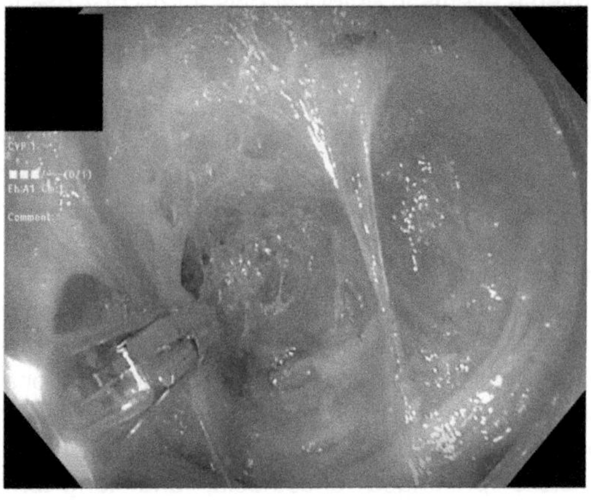

**Fig. 4.** Coagulation grasper on larger submucosal vessel.

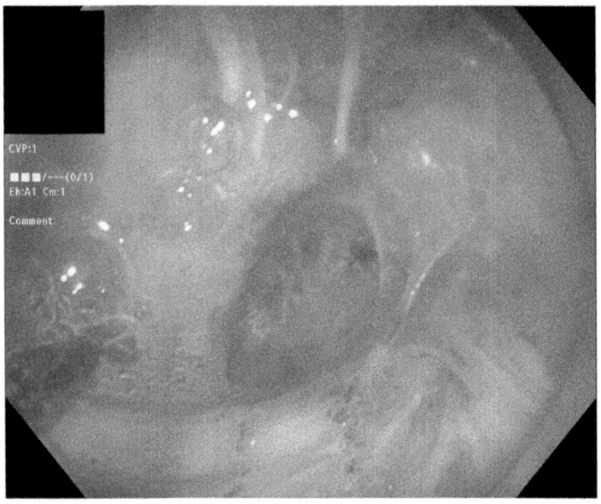

**Fig. 5.** Mucosal staining to confirm distal extent of tunnel.

of foregut pathologic conditions, including the Gastric Peroral Endoscopic Myotomy (G-POEM), Zenker Peroral Endoscopic Myotomy (Z-POEM), and Diverticular Peroral Endoscopic Myotomy (D-POEM).

### *Gastric peroral endoscopic myotomy*

Delayed gastric emptying (DGE) is a chronic condition characterized by pylorus dysfunction often secondary to vagotomy without mechanical obstruction. Clinical manifestations include nausea, vomiting, fullness, bloating, and epigastric pain, which can incur high health care costs. Traditional approaches to DGE include medical management or surgical pyloroplasty or pyloromyotomy. More recently, however, G-POEM has been used as an endoscopic approach to a pyloromyotomy. This procedure involves performing a mucosotomy 5 cm proximal to the pylorus on the lesser curvature of the stomach, short distance submucosal tunneling, and pyloromyotomy using "safe" knives to avoid duodenal injury (Video 2).[16] G-POEM could

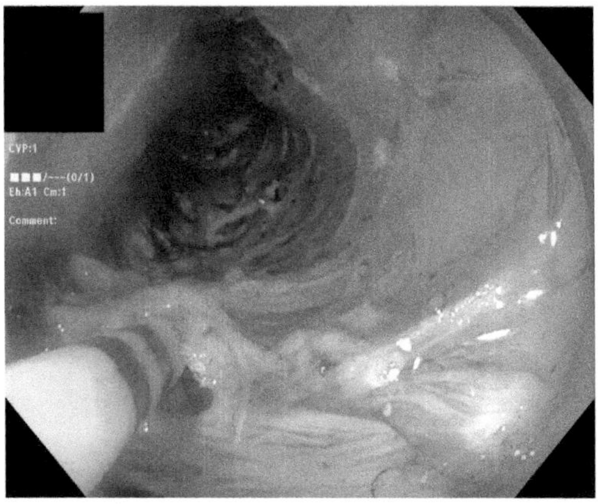

**Fig. 6.** Circular muscle myotomy.

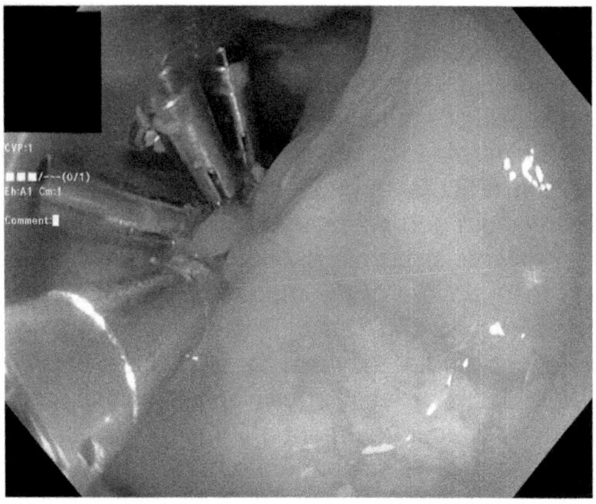

**Fig. 7.** Endoscopic clip closure of mucosotomy.

also potentially be used for gastric conduit outlet obstruction after esophagectomy.

In terms of long-term outcomes compared with other procedural interventions for DGE, G-POEM was shown to be equivalent at 30 and 90 days per Gastroparesis Cardinal Symptom Index (GCSI) and gastric-emptying studies.[17] Additional data supporting the long-term effectiveness of G-POEM include a retrospective case series of 90 patients using the same GCSI score with a clinical response of 85.2% at 1 year of patients who were initial responders to G-POEM.[18]

### *Zenker peroral endoscopic myotomy*

Zenker diverticula are hypopharyngeal pulsion diverticula that can lead to symptoms such as dysphagia, aspiration, malnutrition, or halitosis (**Fig. 8**). The mainstay of treatment has been diverticulectomy via open surgical approach or transoral rigid esophagoscopy with cricopharyngeal myotomy/septotomy.[19] More recently, flexible endoscopic intervention has come onto the scene, such as flexible endoscopic septotomy (FES), initially described in 1995.[20] Since then, a variety

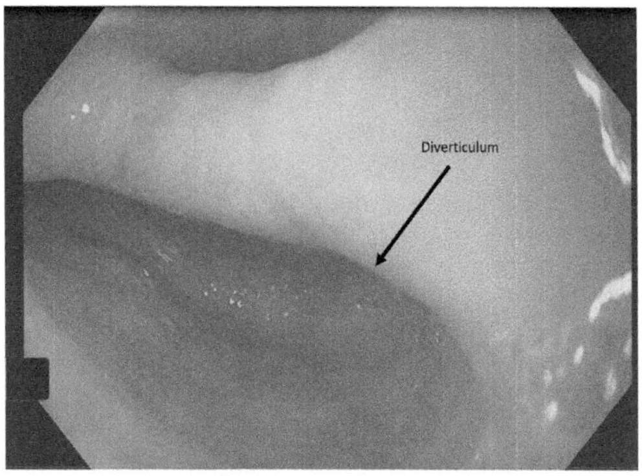


**Fig. 8.** Zenker diverticulum.

of techniques have been developed that are based on the principles of POEM first described by Li and colleagues.[21] This technique involves the creation of a submucosal tunnel in the posterior hypopharynx, tunnel extension to both sides of the muscular septum (**Fig. 9**) through the submucosa of the diverticulum and esophageal true lumen, and cricopharyngeus muscle division (**Figs. 10** and **11**), and then closure of the mucosotomy defect with clips (**Figs. 12** and **13**).[21]

Recent studies have suggested that FES and Z-POEM are at least equivalent, if not superior, to open surgical treatment of Zenker diverticula.[22] In a recent large-scale meta-analysis of available data comparing FES with Z-POEM, higher clinical success was found in patients who underwent Z-POEM (93.0% vs 87.9%). Technical success, adverse events, procedure time, hospital length of stay, and clinical recurrence were similar between FES and Z-POEM.[23] Overall, based on these data, Z-POEM is a comparable, safe, and effective method to treat Zenker diverticula.

### *Diverticular peroral endoscopic myotomy*

After the success of Z-POEM in the management of Zenker diverticula, similar techniques are being used to treat non-Zenker diverticula of the esophagus (D-POEM). Flexible endoscopic septal division (FESD) and rigid endoscopic septotomy have been used for non–Zenker esophageal diverticulum; however, the postprocedural recurrence rate is high (11%–30%).[24] By comparison, several studies have found that the recurrence rate is 11% or less for D-POEM.[25] Failure of FESD has been attributed to incomplete septotomy owing to the fear of perforation. D-POEM allows for a more complete septotomy owing to the protection of the mucosal flap, and the myotomy can be extended distally beyond the diverticulum, similar conceptually to surgical diverticulectomy with myotomy, which prevents recurrence.[25] D-POEM has a significantly higher clinical success rate at 87.07% versus FESD at 75% to 78%.[25]

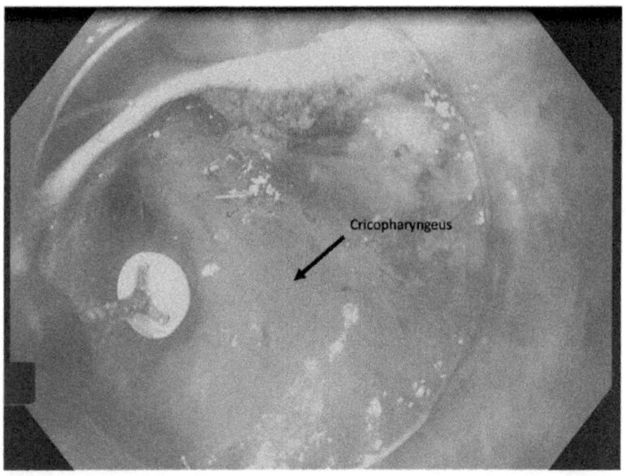


**Fig. 9.** Submucosal dissection isolating the cricopharyngeus muscle.

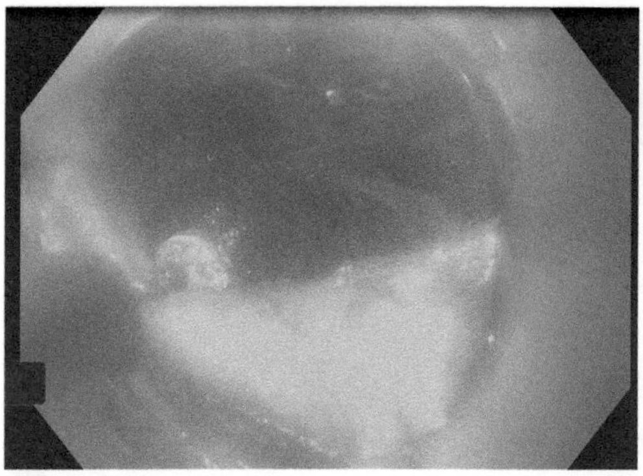

**Fig. 10.** Cricopharyngeus division.

## ADDITIONAL ADVANCED ENDOSCOPIC THERAPIES

### *Endoscopic Stenting*

Several options are available for the palliation of dysphagia related to esophageal cancer and include self-expanding metal stents (SEMS), photodynamic therapy, laser therapy, brachytherapy, and surgical esophageal bypass or diversion.[26–30] SEMS placement has been shown to result in rapid resolution of dysphagia and is recommended for patients with expected short-term survival. Thoracic surgeons should be aware of esophageal stent insertion principles, such as SEMS are preferred over self-expanding plastic stents (SEPS), as they have fewer adverse events and better symptomatic relief, among others.[31,32] Early stent complications include reflux (~10%), pain (~9%), and bleeding (~8%), with late complications of reflux (~15%), pain (~15%), and ingrowth/overgrowth (~14%).[30] No evidence supports differences in outcomes with fully covered

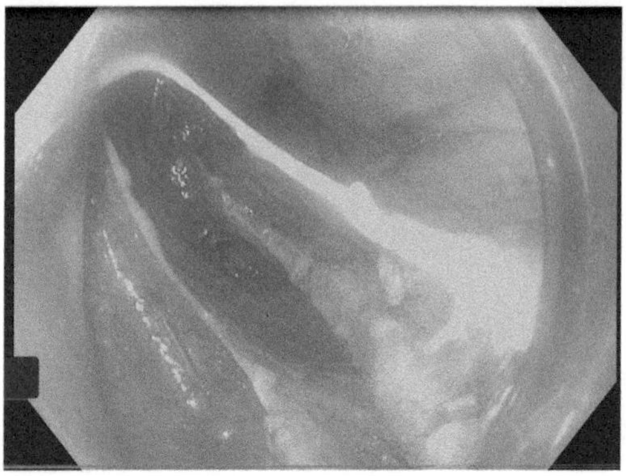

**Fig. 11.** Completed cricopharyngeus division.

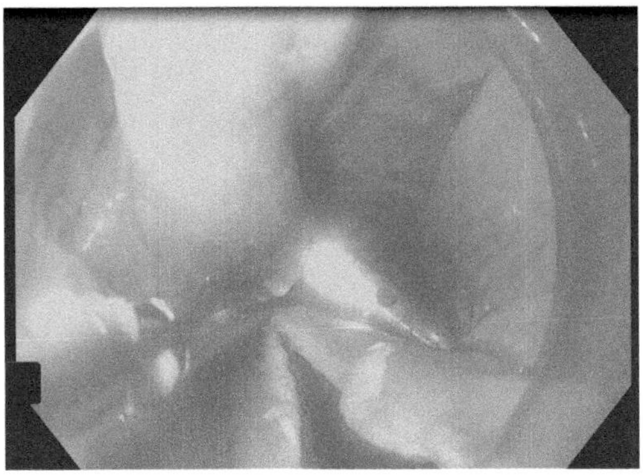

**Fig. 12.** Initial mucosotomy closure.

SEMS versus partially covered SEMS for malignant strictures.[33] In patients who may be expected to have long-term survival, despite taking longer for symptom resolution and needing expertise, brachytherapy may provide more durable relief of symptoms than SEMS.[34,35] Combined brachytherapy and SEMS and irradiated SEMS also hold promise for treating malignant esophageal strictures.[36,37]

Evidence suggests that chemoradiation use before stent placement increases the risk of complications.[38] Some have used stents before neoadjuvant therapy for esophageal cancer to improve dysphagia and nutrition during therapy and before surgery and found significant adverse events and migration during therapy.[39] Biodegradable stents have been used as an alternative in the neoadjuvant setting to avoid SEMS adverse events during treatment. However, 70% of patients required alternative nutritional support despite decreasing dysphagia symptoms.[40] Previously, stent placement before resection was associated with fewer R0 resections, but recent studies have demonstrated no difference in the R0 resection rate or overall complications.[41,42]

SEMS have also been used to treat malignant esophageal fistulas, with success ranging from 56% to 100%, with recurrence of the fistula in 0% to 39%.[30] Stent repositioning or airway stenting in recurrence has been used with some success.[43]

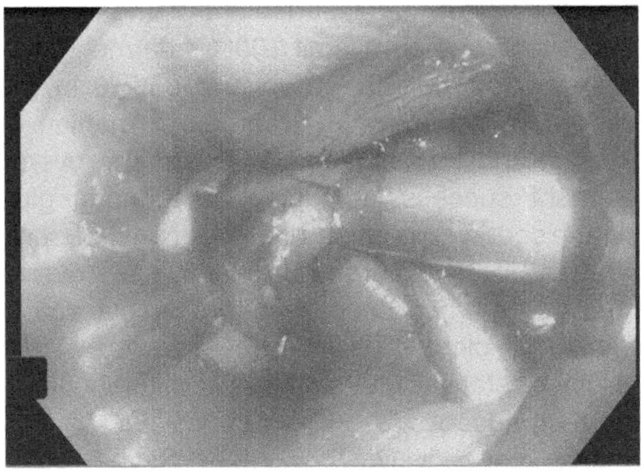

**Fig. 13.** Final mucosotomy closure.

#### *Esophageal stenting for benign disease*

By using their continual expansile force, SEMS have been used for benign esophageal strictures refractory to dilations, with a success rate of approximately 40% and stent migration of 29%.[44] Stent fixation techniques, such as clips or suturing, have decreased the risk of stent migration.[45] SEMS for benign strictures are left in 6 to 8 weeks to allow for remodeling, with longer durations potentially increasing the risk of stent-related complications.[46]

#### *Stents for esophageal perforations*

The success rate of stents for anastomotic leaks/perforations approached 87% regardless of stent type in one multicenter retrospective cohort study.[47] SEMS are preferred over SEPS, given their reduced migration and higher technical success in placement. Clinical prediction models for who may benefit from stent placement have been developed, but these are often complex decisions requiring an individualized approach.[47] Using larger SEMS and suturing the stent have been suggested to decrease stent migration.[48,49] Stent duration is still undecided, and most are removed after 6 to 8 weeks.[50] EVT has also been used to manage postsurgical leaks and has been shown to have a higher closure rate than stents but at the cost of multiple reinterventions.[51] Stents and EVT may be used in conjunction for complex cases.

#### *Esophageal stenting technique*

Most esophageal stents can be safely and effectively placed using a standard flexible upper gastrointestinal (GI) endoscope. The use of fluoroscopy is standard and necessary in most cases, although some endoscopists advocate for deploying stents under direct endoscopic visualization using a pediatric gastroscope in lieu of fluoroscopy. The esophageal stent size is chosen based on the specific details of the esophageal anatomy, characteristics of the stent (such as proximal and distal flared ends), and goals and anticipated duration of stenting. Careful attention must be paid to the proximal and distal landing zones of the stent to ensure appropriate luminal apposition and coverage of the target pathologic condition.

### *Endoluminal Vacuum Therapy*

Although not as expansively studied as esophageal stenting, another approach to esophageal

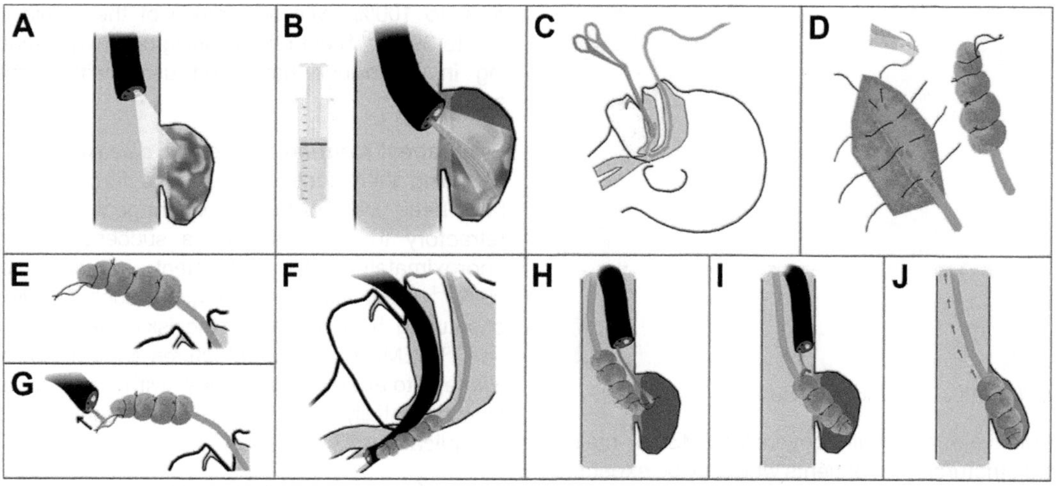


**Fig. 14.** Steps for EVT for esophageal leaks/perforations. (*From* Ooi G, Burton P, Packiyanathan A, et al. Indications and efficacy of endoscopic vacuum-assisted closure therapy for upper gastrointestinal perforations. ANZ J Surg. 2018;88(4):E257-E263.)

perforations or anastomotic leaks includes endoluminal (or endoscopic) vacuum therapy (EVT)/endoscopic vacuum-assisted closure. EVT is based on applying continuous negative pressure to the esophageal defect with a sponge (**Fig. 14**) to drain any persistent infection and accelerate wound healing.[52] Proposed mechanisms of action are similar to those cited when vacuum therapy is applied to nonhealing skin wounds, such as macrodeformation, microdeformation, changes in perfusion, exudate control, and bacterial clearance.[53] In one series of 20 patients with a median fistula size of 1.75 cm, EVT was used for a median of 5 interventions over 14.5 days with a 95% success rate.[54] Those with larger fistulas and patients who underwent neoadjuvant therapy tended to need longer therapy durations. EVT success rates have been echoed in previous studies,[55–57] and a more recent series of upper GI leaks and perforations, the largest with 119 patients, demonstrated clinical success in 71%.[58] In comparison to self-expanding stent placement, EVT has a higher success rate in esophageal leak closure with a pooled odds ratio of 5.51 (95% CI, 2.11–14.88; $P$<.001) as demonstrated in an extensive systematic review and meta-analysis.[59]

Although generally considered safe with a low rate of adverse events, EVT has several drawbacks, including frequent returns to the operating room or endoscopy suite for sponge exchange. Major adverse events are rare; however, there are reservations given the possibility of significant bleeding owing to the possible development of a fistula between the treatment area and major blood vessels.[53] The prior systematic review and meta-analysis showed a lower major complication rate than endoscopic stenting ($P$ = .011)[59]; however, several small studies have documented deaths from significant hemorrhage associated with EVT. One small (n = 52) prospective study had 2 EVT-associated deaths from acute hemorrhage,[57] and another retrospective study (n = 21) had 2 bleeding events, which were subsequently managed with aortic stenting.[60] Adverse events can be avoided if care is taken to closely monitor EVT output, to perform timely and atraumatic sponge exchanges, and to act upon signs of hemorrhage early.

### *Endoscopic Internal Drainage*

As an alternative to EVT, endoscopic internal drainage (EID) has been proposed to manage anastomotic leaks following oncologic upper GI surgery. EID involves endoscopically guided placement of a pigtail catheter into extraluminal collections to allow for passive drainage into the GI tract.[61] In a retrospective study comparing EID with EVT for the management of anastomotic leaks, there was an overall 100% treatment success rate for the EID group and 85.2% in the EVT group; however, EID required a median of 42 days, and EVT required 17 days. The overall treatment success included placing fibrin glue over the scope clips and an SEMS for final closure. Although EID had a statistically significant overall improved treatment success before the placement of final leak closure devices, EID versus EVT did not have statistically significant differences in treatment success (91.4% vs 74.1%, EID vs EVT groups, respectively; $P$ = .09). Nevertheless, larger-scale studies with a more generous range of anastomotic defect sizes are necessary before EID can be recommended as a standard approach to treating esophageal perforations or anastomotic leaks.

### *Endoscopic Suturing and Clipping*

In addition to EVT and stenting, endoscopic suturing or clipping can be a means to manage small GI leaks or perforations. Two varieties of clips exist to manage small defects: through-the-scope (TTS) and over-the-scope (OTS). TTS clips can be used to close chronic fistulae and leaks; however, given the limited pressure that can be applied and the tendency to dislodge,[62] there is debate over the effectiveness of this intervention in more chronic leaks or fistula with an effectiveness rate ranging from 59% to 83%.[63,64] OTS clips, on the other hand, allow for a larger defect closure with a stronger closing force.[65] OTS has a higher success rate with treating anastomotic leaks than chronic fistulae,[62] with one systematic review study demonstrating a success rate of 66% for anastomotic leaks and 51.5% for fistulae.[66] Anecdotally, the authors of this review have found both TTS and OTS clips suboptimal for all but relatively small and fresh perforations, as the clips perform poorly on friable tissue. Furthermore, great care must be taken in deploying the OTS clips, as these can catch tissue external to the esophagus and may lead to aerodigestive or vascular fistulae in rare, but potentially catastrophic complications.

For the advanced endoscopist, endoscopic suturing systems also exist to assist in closure of GI defects. The OverStitch (Apollo Endosurgery, Austin, TX, USA) uses a double therapeutic channel endoscope and allows continuous suturing.[62] Limited data exist on applying this technology to esophageal anastomotic leak and fistula management. Long-term data show a successful closure rate of fistulae between 40% and 80%[67,68] and a low rate of leak closure (27%).[67] To improve the clinical success rate, one single-center case series used the OverStitch in conjunction with SEMS placement and anchoring. They observed a clinical success rate of 77% without stent placement and anchoring. With the addition of stent placement and anchoring, the success rate improved to 85%. This study was limited because treatment modalities were divided by tissue quality before repair and small sample size. Although OverStitch offers a promising modality for defect closure, the overall long-term success rate currently is low, most likely owing to the requirement of high technical proficiency with the device and appropriate patient selection, which requires further research.

## FUTURE DIRECTIONS

One can imagine future improvements in current technologies, such as stents, clips, and suturing, as well as new technologies to address novel approaches to the pathologic conditions discussed above and their postprocedural complications. One such example is endoscopic solutions to significant GERD after POEM. A single-session endoscopic fundoplication has been proposed after peroral endoscopic myotomy (POEM + F). Early data show excellent short-term outcomes in controlling post-POEM gastroesophageal reflux while adding 46.7 minutes to the procedure time.[69]

As robotic-assisted surgery becomes more ubiquitous across the country, some have explored the possibility of adapting this platform to endoscopic surgery. As robotic-assisted surgery is primarily being developed for diagnostic purposes, several advances have been made to robotize advanced therapeutic procedures. One limitation of current techniques is that the operator is responsible for directing the endoscope. At the same time, the assistant is responsible for the insertion, removal, and manipulation of the instrumentation to perform the procedure. Ruiter and colleagues[70] proposed a platform that allows one-handed manipulation of an endoscope, leaving the other hand available for manipulation of instrumentation. In addition, although robotic-assisted technologies are primarily available for lower endoscopy applications, few groups have endeavored to apply robotic-assisted technologies to upper endoscopic procedures. The Via-Cath system is one such innovation from Berlin, Germany, that functions similarly to traditional teleoperated robots with long-shafted instruments that function through an endoscope with a flexible overtube. This system is currently in the very early stages of development.[71] The MASTER (Master And Slave Transluminal Endoscopic Robot) is similar in terms of current procedural endoscopy, requiring 2 individuals to operate together, one with the instrumentation and the other with the endoscope. The advantages of this platform allow for greater dexterity and haptic feedback.[72] Other platforms include i2Snake[73] and K-FLEX,[74] which are variations on the theme of flexible manipulators integrated into traditional endoscopes to allow for greater instrument and camera manipulation. One can imagine that improved endoscopic robotic technology could increase the indications for endoscopic resection of gastroesophageal malignancies especially if allowing for an endoscopic transluminal lymphadenectomy in conjunction with EMR, ESD, or full-thickness resection and closure.

In addition, endoscopic drug delivery has been described, as the GI tract involves a large surface that allows for increased local and systemic drug levels and mitigates first-pass metabolism of drugs. Methods that have been proposed include needle injection, jetting, iontophoresis (passing an electrical current through the mucosa), ultrasound, hyperthermia, magnetic, and convection.[75]

Finally, artificial intelligence (AI) algorithms have been applied to various industries to optimize machine performance. The medical industry is no exception, and the hope is that with ongoing research, endoscopic procedures' time, cost, and efficacy can be improved with this technology. In addition to the utility of AI for diagnostic endoscopy, there is early research into the application of AI aiding in procedures such as POEM and PD. For example, an early feasibility study by Ebigbo and colleagues[76] demonstrated that with visual data sets, their algorithm could detect structures, such as vessels, the submucosa, and muscularis, and identify instruments within the visual field. Future directions include training the AI system with more samples and the ability to use the detection system during procedures for real-time feedback and even to help guide the proper dissection plane.

## SUMMARY

The thoracic surgeon, well-versed in advanced endoscopic techniques, can offer various therapeutic options for the primary treatment of foregut pathologic condition as well as for complication management. For example, POEM has been demonstrated to be a noninferior, safe option for treating achalasia and POEM variations effective for treating several other gastroesophageal pathologic conditions. The endoscopic management of esophageal leaks and perforations also continues to evolve, with stents, clips, suturing, EVT, and EID all holding promise for treating this challenging clinical problem. These endoscopic options may have less risk of adverse events compared with traditional operative interventions, particularly for poor surgical candidates. In addition, having experience with both endoscopic and operative interventions for these diseases allows the surgeon to maintain equipoise and properly engage in the shared decision-making process with patients when choosing interventions. As endoscopic technology continues to advance, thoracic surgeons should be at the forefront of these new technologies, helping to drive innovations in a safe and evidence-based manner in this rapidly expanding field.

## CLINICS CARE POINTS

- Achalasia treatment is evolving, with peroral endoscopic myotomy demonstrating noninferiority to traditional surgical myotomy in terms of dysphagia but with increased rates of reflux. This may be a good option for many patients, especially symptomatic patients deemed high risk for surgical intervention.
- Variations of peroral endoscopic myotomy, such as Gastric Peroral Endoscopic Myotomy, Zenker Peroral Endoscopic Myotomy, and Diverticular Peroral Endoscopic Myotomy, are evolving techniques and are also proving effective compared with their surgical alternatives
- Additional endoscopic therapies for the thoracic surgeon include endoscopic stenting for esophageal cancer palliation, malignant fistulas, benign esophageal strictures, and anastomotic leaks/perforations. Endoluminal vacuum therapy, endoscopic internal drainage, and endoscopic suturing/clipping are additional therapies available to the thoracic surgeon for upper gastrointestinal leaks and perforations.
- Improvements in stenting, clips, and suturing can be expected as well as possible future endoscopic reflux management in peroral endoscopic myotomy, robotic advancement of endoscopic surgical capabilities, and artificial intelligence augmentation of procedures.
- Endoscopic treatments are rapidly advancing, and the thoracic surgeon should acquire these skills in lockstep.

## DISCLOSURE

The authors have nothing to disclose.

## SUPPLEMENTARY DATA

Supplementary data related to this article can be found online at https://doi.org/10.1016/j.thorsurg.2023.04.015.

## REFERENCES

1. Fanelli RD, Sultany MS. Surgeons performing endoscopy: why, how, and when? Ann Laparosc Endosc Surg 2019;4:66.
2. Fukami N. Endoscopic Submucosal Dissection in the Esophagus: Indications, Techniques, and Outcomes. Gastrointest Endosc Clin N Am 2023;33(1):55–66.
3. Organs of the chest cavity. In: Paulsen F, Waschke J, Sobotta J, editors. Sobotta Atlas of human anatomy.

2: internal Organs. 16th edition. Munich (Germany): Elsevier; 2018. p. 18. English version with Latin nomenclature.
4. Kahrilas PJ, Bredenoord AJ, Fox M, et al. The Chicago Classification of esophageal motility disorders, v3.0. Neuro Gastroenterol Motil 2015;27(2):160–74.
5. Townsend CM. Sabiston textbook of surgery : the biological basis of modern surgical practice. 21st edition. St. Louis (MO): Elsevier; 2022. p. 2147. xxviii.
6. Inoue H, Minami H, Kobayashi Y, et al. Peroral endoscopic myotomy (POEM) for esophageal achalasia. Endoscopy 2010;42(4):265–71.
7. Eckardt AJ, Eckardt VF. Treatment and surveillance strategies in achalasia: an update. Nat Rev Gastroenterol Hepatol 2011;8(6):311–9.
8. Dirks RC, Kohn GP, Slater B, et al. Is peroral endoscopic myotomy (POEM) more effective than pneumatic dilation and Heller myotomy? A systematic review and meta-analysis. Surg Endosc 2021; 35(5):1949–62.
9. Schlottmann F, Luckett DJ, Fine J, et al. Laparoscopic Heller Myotomy Versus Peroral Endoscopic Myotomy (POEM) for Achalasia: A Systematic Review and Meta-analysis. Ann Surg 2018;267(3): 451–60.
10. de Moura ETH, Jukemura J, Ribeiro IB, et al. Peroral endoscopic myotomy vs laparoscopic myotomy and partial fundoplication for esophageal achalasia: A single-center randomized controlled trial. World J Gastroenterol 2022;28(33):4875–89.
11. Werner YB, Hakanson B, Martinek J, et al. Endoscopic or Surgical Myotomy in Patients with Idiopathic Achalasia. N Engl J Med 2019;381(23): 2219–29.
12. Simkova D, Mares J, Vackova Z, et al. Periprocedural safety profile of peroral endoscopic myotomy (POEM)-a retrospective analysis of adverse events according to two different classifications. Surg Endosc 2022. https://doi.org/10.1007/s00464-022-09621-z.
13. Haito-Chavez Y, Inoue H, Beard KW, et al. Comprehensive Analysis of Adverse Events Associated With Per Oral Endoscopic Myotomy in 1826 Patients: An International Multicenter Study. Am J Gastroenterol 2017;112(8):1267–76.
14. Liu X, Yao L, Cheng J, et al. Landscape of Adverse Events Related to Peroral Endoscopic Myotomy in 3135 Patients and a Risk-Scoring System to Predict Major Adverse Events. Clin Gastroenterol Hepatol 2021;19(9):1959–1966 e3.
15. Servais E. Per-oral endoscopic myotomy (POEM). 2021. 11/6/2022. Available at: https://www.youtube.com/watch?v=7cOi-_EVNa0. Accessed December 15, 2022.
16. Parsa N, Friedel D, Stavropoulos SN. POEM, GPOEM, and ZPOEM. Dig Dis Sci 2022;67(5): 1500–20.
17. Landreneau JP, Strong AT, El-Hayek K, et al. Laparoscopic pyloroplasty versus endoscopic per-oral pyloromyotomy for the treatment of gastroparesis. Surg Endosc 2019;33(3):773–81.
18. Abdelfatah MM, Noll A, Kapil N, et al. Long-term Outcome of Gastric Per-Oral Endoscopic Pyloromyotomy in Treatment of Gastroparesis. Clin Gastroenterol Hepatol 2021;19(4):816–24.
19. Johnson CM, Postma GN. Zenker Diverticulum–Which Surgical Approach Is Superior? JAMA Otolaryngol Head Neck Surg 2016;142(4):401–3.
20. Mulder CJ, den Hartog G, Robijn RJ, et al. Flexible endoscopic treatment of Zenker's diverticulum: a new approach. Endoscopy 1995;27(6):438–42.
21. Li QL, Chen WF, Zhang XC, et al. Submucosal Tunneling Endoscopic Septum Division: A Novel Technique for Treating Zenker's Diverticulum. Gastroenterology 2016;151(6):1071–4.
22. Weusten B, Barret M, Bredenoord AJ, et al. Endoscopic management of gastrointestinal motility disorders - part 2: European Society of Gastrointestinal Endoscopy (ESGE) Guideline. Endoscopy 2020; 52(7):600–14.
23. Zhang H, Huang S, Xia H, et al. The role of peroral endoscopic myotomy for Zenker's diverticulum: a systematic review and meta-analysis. Surg Endosc 2022;36(5):2749–59.
24. Ishaq S, Siau K, Kuwai T, et al. Zenker's peroral endoscopic myotomy (Z-POEM) for recurrent Zenker diverticulum: not so fast. Endoscopy 2021; 53(7):767.
25. Mandavdhare HS, Praveen Kumar M, Jha D, et al. Diverticular per oral endoscopic myotomy (DPOEM) for esophageal diverticular disease: a systematic review and meta-analysis. Esophagus 2021;18(3): 436–50.
26. Alderson D, Wright PD. Laser recanalization versus endoscopic intubation in the palliation of malignant dysphagia. Br J Surg 1990;77(10):1151–3.
27. Aoki T, Osaka Y, Takagi Y, et al. Comparative study of self-expandable metallic stent and bypass surgery for inoperable esophageal cancer. Dis Esophagus 2001;14(3–4):208–11.
28. Bergquist H, Wenger U, Johnsson E, et al. Stent insertion or endoluminal brachytherapy as palliation of patients with advanced cancer of the esophagus and gastroesophageal junction. Results of a randomized, controlled clinical trial. Dis Esophagus 2005;18(3):131–9.
29. Yoon HY, Cheon YK, Choi HJ, et al. Role of Photodynamic Therapy in the Palliation of Obstructing Esophageal Cancer. Kor J Intern Med 2012;27(3):278.
30. Spaander MCW, Van Der Bogt RD, Baron TH, et al. Esophageal stenting for benign and malignant disease: European Society of Gastrointestinal Endoscopy (ESGE) Guideline – Update 2021. Endoscopy 2021;53(07):751–62.

31. Dai Y, Li C, Xie Y, et al. Interventions for dysphagia in oesophageal cancer. Cochrane Database Syst Rev 2014;2014(10):Cd005048.
32. Qayed E, Anand GS, Aihara H, et al. Core curriculum for endoluminal stent placement. Gastrointest Endosc 2020;92(3):463–8.
33. Didden P, Reijm AN, Erler NS, et al. Fully vs. partially covered selfexpandable metal stent for palliation of malignant esophageal strictures: a randomized trial (the COPAC study). Endoscopy 2018;50(10): 961–71.
34. Fuccio L, Mandolesi D, Farioli A, et al. Brachytherapy for the palliation of dysphagia owing to esophageal cancer: A systematic review and meta-analysis of prospective studies. Radiother Oncol 2017; 122(3):332–9.
35. Homs MY, Steyerberg EW, Eijkenboom WM, et al. Single-dose brachytherapy versus metal stent placement for the palliation of dysphagia from oesophageal cancer: multicentre randomised trial. Lancet 2004;364(9444):1497–504.
36. Bergquist H, Johnsson E, Nyman J, et al. Combined stent insertion and single high-dose brachytherapy in patients with advanced esophageal cancer–results of a prospective safety study. Dis Esophagus 2012;25(5):410–5.
37. Chen HL, Shen WQ, Liu K. Radioactive self-expanding stents for palliative management of unresectable esophageal cancer: a systematic review and meta-analysis. Dis Esophagus 2017;30(5):1–16.
38. Reijm AN, Didden P, Schelling SJC, et al. Self-expandable metal stent placement for malignant esophageal strictures - changes in clinical outcomes over time. Endoscopy 2019;51(1):18–29.
39. Nagaraja V, Cox MR, Eslick GD. Safety and efficacy of esophageal stents preceding or during neoadjuvant chemotherapy for esophageal cancer: a systematic review and meta-analysis. J Gastrointest Oncol 2014;5(2):119–26.
40. van den Berg MW, Walter D, de Vries EM, et al. Biodegradable stent placement before neoadjuvant chemoradiotherapy as a bridge to surgery in patients with locally advanced esophageal cancer. Gastrointest Endosc 2014;80(5):908–13.
41. Mariette C, Gronnier C, Duhamel A, et al. Self-expanding covered metallic stent as a bridge to surgery in esophageal cancer: impact on oncologic outcomes. J Am Coll Surg 2015;220(3):287–96.
42. Rodrigues-Pinto E, Ferreira-Silva J, Sousa-Pinto B, et al. Self-expandable metal stents in esophageal cancer before preoperative neoadjuvant therapy: efficacy, safety, and long-term outcomes. Surg Endosc 2021;35(9):5130–9.
43. Włodarczyk JR, Kużdżał J. Safety and efficacy of airway stenting in patients with malignant oesophago-airway fistula. J Thorac Dis 2018;10(5):2731–9.
44. Fuccio L, Hassan C, Frazzoni L, et al. Clinical outcomes following stent placement in refractory benign esophageal stricture: a systematic review and meta-analysis. Endoscopy 2016;48(2):141–8.
45. Law R, Prabhu A, Fujii-Lau L, et al. Stent migration following endoscopic suture fixation of esophageal self-expandable metal stents: a systematic review and meta-analysis. Surg Endosc 2018;32(2): 675–81.
46. van Halsema EE, Wong K, Song LM, et al. Safety of endoscopic removal of self-expandable stents after treatment of benign esophageal diseases. Gastrointest Endosc 2013;77(1):18–28.
47. van Halsema EE, Kappelle WFW, Weusten B, et al. Stent placement for benign esophageal leaks, perforations, and fistulae: a clinical prediction rule for successful leakage control. Endoscopy 2018;50(2): 98–108.
48. Rodrigues-Pinto E, Pereira P, Sousa-Pinto B, et al. Retrospective multicenter study on endoscopic treatment of upper GI postsurgical leaks. Gastrointest Endosc 2021;93(6):1283–99.e2.
49. Ngamruengphong S, Sharaiha R, Sethi A, et al. Fully-covered metal stents with endoscopic suturing vs. partially-covered metal stents for benign upper gastrointestinal diseases: a comparative study. Endosc Int Open 2018;6(2):E217–23.
50. Kamarajah SK, Bundred J, Spence G, et al. Critical Appraisal of the Impact of Oesophageal Stents in the Management of Oesophageal Anastomotic Leaks and Benign Oesophageal Perforations: An Updated Systematic Review. World J Surg 2020; 44(4):1173–89.
51. Scognamiglio P, Reeh M, Karstens K, et al. Endoscopic vacuum therapy versus stenting for postoperative esophago-enteric anastomotic leakage: systematic review and meta-analysis. Endoscopy 2020;52(8):632–42.
52. Moore CB, Almoghrabi O, Hofstetter W, et al. Endoluminal wound vac: an evolving role in treatment of esophageal perforation. J Vis Surg 2020;6:43.
53. de Moura DTH, de Moura B, Manfredi MA, et al. Role of endoscopic vacuum therapy in the management of gastrointestinal transmural defects. World J Gastrointest Endosc 2019;11(5):329–44.
54. Min YW, Kim T, Lee H, et al. Endoscopic vacuum therapy for postoperative esophageal leak. BMC Surg 2019;19(1). https://doi.org/10.1186/s12893-019-0497-5.
55. Brangewitz M, Voigtländer T, Helfritz FA, et al. Endoscopic closure of esophageal intrathoracic leaks: stent versus endoscopic vacuum-assisted closure, a retrospective analysis. Endoscopy 2013;45(6):433–8.
56. Schorsch T, Müller C, Loske G. [Endoscopic vacuum therapy of perforations and anastomotic insufficiency of the esophagus]. Chirurg 2014;85(12):

1081–93. Endoskopische Vakuumtherapie von Perforationen und Anastomoseninsuffizienzen des Ösophagus.
57. Laukoetter MG, Mennigen R, Neumann PA, et al. Successful closure of defects in the upper gastrointestinal tract by endoscopic vacuum therapy (EVT): a prospective cohort study. Surg Endosc 2017; 31(6):2687–96.
58. Jung DH, Huh CW, Min YW, et al. Endoscopic vacuum therapy for the management of upper GI leaks and perforations: a multicenter retrospective study of factors associated with treatment failure (with video). Gastrointest Endosc 2022;95(2):281–90.
59. Rausa E, Asti E, Aiolfi A, et al. Comparison of endoscopic vacuum therapy versus endoscopic stenting for esophageal leaks: systematic review and meta-analysis. Dis Esophagus 2018;31(11). https://doi.org/10.1093/dote/doy060.
60. Pournaras DJ, Hardwick RH, Safranek PM, et al. Endoluminal Vacuum Therapy (E-Vac): A Treatment Option in Oesophagogastric Surgery. World J Surg 2018;42(8):2507–11.
61. Jung CFM, Hallit R, Müller-Dornieden A, et al. Endoscopic internal drainage and low negative-pressure endoscopic vacuum therapy for anastomotic leaks after oncologic upper gastrointestinal surgery. Endoscopy 2022;54(1):71–4.
62. Cereatti F, Grassia R, Drago A, et al. Endoscopic management of gastrointestinal leaks and fistulae: What option do we have? World J Gastroenterol 2020;26(29):4198–217.
63. Magdeburg R, Collet P, Post S, et al. Endoclipping of iatrogenic colonic perforation to avoid surgery. Surg Endosc 2008;22(6):1500–4.
64. Cho SB, Lee WS, Joo YE, et al. Therapeutic options for iatrogenic colon perforation: feasibility of endoscopic clip closure and predictors of the need for early surgery. Surg Endosc 2012;26(2):473–9.
65. Watkins JR, Farivar AS. Endoluminal Therapies for Esophageal Perforations and Leaks. Thorac Surg Clin 2018;28(4):541–54.
66. Kobara H, Mori H, Nishiyama N, et al. Over-the-scope clip system: A review of 1517 cases over 9 years. J Gastroenterol Hepatol 2019;34(1):22–30.
67. Sharaiha RZ, Kumta NA, DeFilippis EM, et al. A Large Multicenter Experience With Endoscopic Suturing for Management of Gastrointestinal Defects and Stent Anchorage in 122 Patients: A Retrospective Review. J Clin Gastroenterol 2016;50(5):388–92.
68. Mukewar S, Kumar N, Catalano M, et al. Safety and efficacy of fistula closure by endoscopic suturing: a multi-center study. Endoscopy 2016;48(11):1023–8.
69. Bapaye A, Dashatwar P, Dharamsi S, et al. Single-session endoscopic fundoplication after peroral endoscopic myotomy (POEM+F) for prevention of post gastroesophageal reflux - 1-year follow-up study. Endoscopy 2021;53(11):1114–21.
70. Ruiter JG, Bonnema GM, van der Voort MC, et al. Robotic control of a traditional flexible endoscope for therapy. J Robot Surg 2013;7(3):227–34.
71. Peters BS, Armijo PR, Krause C, et al. Review of emerging surgical robotic technology. Surg Endosc 2018;32(4):1636–55.
72. Yeung BP, Gourlay T. A technical review of flexible endoscopic multitasking platforms. Int J Surg 2012;10(7):345–54.
73. Berthet-Rayne P, Gras G, Leibrandt K, et al. The i(2) Snake Robotic Platform for Endoscopic Surgery. Ann Biomed Eng 2018;46(10):1663–75.
74. Hwang M, Kwon DS, FLEX K-. A flexible robotic platform for scar-free endoscopic surgery. Int J Med Robot 2020;16(2):e2078.
75. Byrne J, Huang HW, McRae JC, et al. Devices for drug delivery in the gastrointestinal tract: A review of systems physically interacting with the mucosa for enhanced delivery. Adv Drug Deliv Rev 2021; 177:113926.
76. Ebigbo A, Mendel R, Scheppach MW, et al. Vessel and tissue recognition during third-space endoscopy using a deep learning algorithm. Gut 2022; 71(12):2388–90.

# Technical Aspects of Robotic First Rib Resection

Matthew R.L. Egyud, MD[a], Scott Holmes, CMI[b], Bryan M. Burt, MD[a,*]

**KEYWORDS**

- Thoracic outlet syndrome • First rib resection • Chest wall resection
- Robotic video-assisted thoracoscopic surgery

**KEY POINTS**

- First rib resection and scalenectomy (FRR) is the surgical treatment of thoracic outlet syndrome.
- The transthoracic robotic approach to FRR provides outstanding exposure of thoracic outlet.
- Transthoracic FRR allows conduct of the operation without retraction of neurovascular structures.
- The transthoracic robotic approach minimizes the morbidity associated with FRR.

## INTRODUCTION

Thoracic outlet syndrome (TOS) is a trio of conditions resulting from compression of the neurovascular structures of the upper extremity. Each of these compressions, brachial plexus causing neurogenic TOS (NTOS), the subclavian vein causing venous TOS (VTOS), and the subclavian artery causing arterial TOS (ATOS), has a unique clinical presentation. NTOS presents with pain, paresthesias, and weakness of the upper extremity with overhead activity progressing to rest symptoms. VTOS presents with acute upper extremity venous thrombosis (Paget–Schroetter syndrome) or positional edema and swelling without thrombosis (McCleery syndrome). ATOS presents with chronic claudication, pallor, and pain or acute limb-threating thrombosis. Resection of the first rib and scalene muscles is the surgical treatment of TOS.

### *Surgical Anatomy*

The thoracic outlet is located at the intersection of the neck and the chest and through it runs the brachial plexus and subclavian artery and vein as they enter or exit the upper extremity. The brachial plexus and subclavian artery enter the upper extremity by traversing the scalene triangle, a space bordered anteriorly by the anterior scalene muscle, posteriorly by the middle scalene muscle, and inferiorly by the first rib. The subclavian vein enters the thorax from the upper extremity through costoclavicular space, a space bordered anteriorly by the anterior scalene muscle, medially by the subclavius muscle and costoclavicular ligament, inferiorly by the first rib, and superficially by the clavicle. Muscular hypertrophy plus congenital anatomic variations result in dynamic compression of neurovascular structures. Individuals performing repetitive upper extremity motions, such as assembly line workers, construction workers, and athletes such as swimmers, baseball pitchers, and tennis players, are particularly prone to the muscular hypertrophy causing repetitive compression that precipitates symptoms.[1] Cervical ribs or elongated T7 transverse processes and associated fibromuscular bands to the first rib are important congenital variants that predispose to brachial plexus compression and are seen approximately 5% to 9% of patients.[2,3]

#### *First rib resection*

First rib resection and scalenectomy (FRR) has historically been performed through open supraclavicular and transaxillary approaches that have inherent exposure limitations and require

[a] Division of Thoracic Surgery, The Michael E. Debakey Department of Surgery, Baylor College of Medicine, One Baylor Plaza, Houston, TX 77030, USA; [b] The Michael E. Debakey Department of Surgery, Baylor College of Medicine, Houston, TX, USA
* Corresponding author.
*E-mail address:* Bryan.Burt@bcm.edu

Thorac Surg Clin 33 (2023) 265–271
https://doi.org/10.1016/j.thorsurg.2023.04.005

manipulation and/or retraction of neurovascular structures that can result in operative morbidity. Herein, we describe technical considerations for the robotic transthoracic approach to FRR that overcomes these limitations and that allows conduct of the operation without retraction of the brachial plexus, subclavian artery and vein, and phrenic nerve. Compared with the traditional open approaches, a transthoracic robotic approach to FRR permits near complete exposure of the first rib and conduct of the operation without manipulation of neurovascular structures, which we have found to improve operative safety.[4] Whereas both video-assisted thoracoscopic and robot-assisted thoracoscopic techniques are available, we prefer the robotic approach due to a high-definition visibility of the operative field and greater precision of surgical instrumentation.[5]

**Operative technique of robotic first rib resection**

***Preoperative considerations*** A thorough diagnostic TOS workup should be performed. Patients should have sufficient pulmonary reserve to tolerate single-lung ventilation. Data from the Disability of the Arm, Hand, and Shoulder questionnaire, visual analog scale for pain, or other questionnaires can be collected before and after surgery as a patient-reported metric to understand surgical outcomes.

***Instrumentation*** We use the DaVinci Xi platform. Instruments include.

- Three 8-mm robotic ports
- One 10-mm assistant port
- 8 mm 0° camera, though a 30° camera can be used
- Prograsp forceps
- Hook monopolar energy instrument
- Curved bipolar dissector
- Handheld suction irrigator
- An electric drill such as the Medtronic Midasrex
- Thoracoscopic ring forceps

***Positioning and marking*** After induction of anesthesia, a double-lumen endotracheal tube or bronchial blocker is placed to achieve single-lung isolation. Neuromuscular blockade with an agent like rocuronium or vecuronium is preferred. The patient is positioned in full lateral decubitus position with the arm abducted 90° and flexion point of the bed at the level of the xiphoid. The bed is flexed.

The scapular borders are marked for reference. The general positions of the three 8-mm robotic ports and assistant ports are marked (**Fig. 1**). The first marking is the posterior 8 mm port, which is marked just behind the scapular tip. This generally corresponds to the fifth or sixth intercostal space. The correct placement of this port is critical, as the drill will be introduced though this port later and should have a straight trajectory toward its targets of the posterior and anterior first rib. The anterior 8-mm port is marked around the midclavicular line in the general area of the third or fourth intercostal space. The difference is split and the 8 mm camera port marking is made around midaxillary line at the level of the seventh intercostal space. The assistant port marking is made around the ninth intercostal space in the anterior axillary line. The field is prepped and draped.

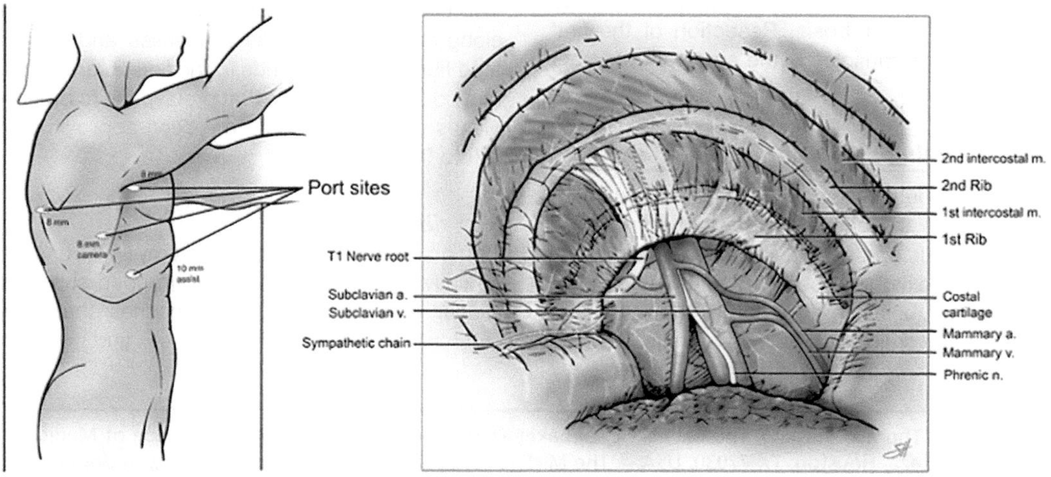


**Fig. 1.** Port placement and survey of anatomy (*right chest*). Three 8-mm robotic ports and a 10-mm assistant ports are used. The transthoracic exposure afforded by the robotic platform permits exceptional visualization of the entirety of the first rib and neurovascular structures. (Illustration by Scott Holmes. CMI, copyright Baylor College of Medicine.)

***Port placement*** The camera port is introduced, the camera is inserted, and capnothorax with 8 mm of Hg of insufflation is achieved. Dilute marcaine is placed subpleurally in the fourth through ninth interspaces, posteriorly, for rib blocks. The two additional robotic ports are then placed under direct vision. The 10-mm assistant port is placed. Three arms of the robot are docked and the first rib is targeted. A grasper such as a Prograsp forcep is inserted into the posterior working port, and energized dissection tool such as the hook cautery is inserted into the anterior port. The complete anatomic survey of the thoracic outlet is then performed.

***Survey of anatomy*** The first rib, second rib, first intercostal muscle, and the costal cartilage are identified. The T1 nerve root, which traces into the brachial plexus, and the phrenic nerve are identified. An accessory phrenic nerve is present in an intrathoracic location in approximately 40% of patients, and its presence or absence is understood. The subclavian artery and vein are identified, as are the mammary artery and vein (see **Fig. 1**).

***First intercostal muscle and pleural dissection*** The hook energy device is used to separate the first intercostal muscle from the lateral aspect of the first rib. The surgeon can use the bony edge of the first rib as a landmark to complete this dissection anteriorly and posteriorly. The parietal pleura is then swept off of the medial aspect of the first rib using the hook dissector with blunt dissection and point energy (**Fig. 2**). Soft tissue dissection proceeds anteriorly, and the costochondral junction is dissected just medial to the mammary artery and vein.

***Division of the first rib*** Once dissected, the cartilage at the anterior portion of the rib can typically be divided at the costoclavicular junction using energy from hook cautery (**Fig. 3**). The assistant removes the resultant opaque smoke from the field using the suction irrigator. Occasionally, ossification of the costal cartilage limits complete division at this time, and this will be treated mechanically with the drill, later. The curved bipolar dissector is then introduced and the posterior aspect of the first intercostal muscle dissection is completed, caring to protect the T1 nerve root. The soft tissue at the very medial aspect of the first rib is dissected using precise bipolar energy after sweeping the pleura completely off of the medial rib. The joint between the first rib and the transverse process can often be entered and partially dissected.

The posterior rib is now divided mechanically with a drill, operated thoracoscopically. The posterior arm of the robot is de-docked, and the posterior port is removed. A drill is inserted through the posterior incision and an assistant places a suction irrigator from the assistant port and can protect the T1 nerve root. From the robotic console, zoom is applied at 2x to allow for improved vision of the section of the rib to divide while minimizing the risk of debris contacting the camera and distorting visualization. The drill is activated and the assistant paints the rib with occasional irrigation for both visualization and cooling (**Fig. 4**). The posterior rib is divided at the level of the transverse

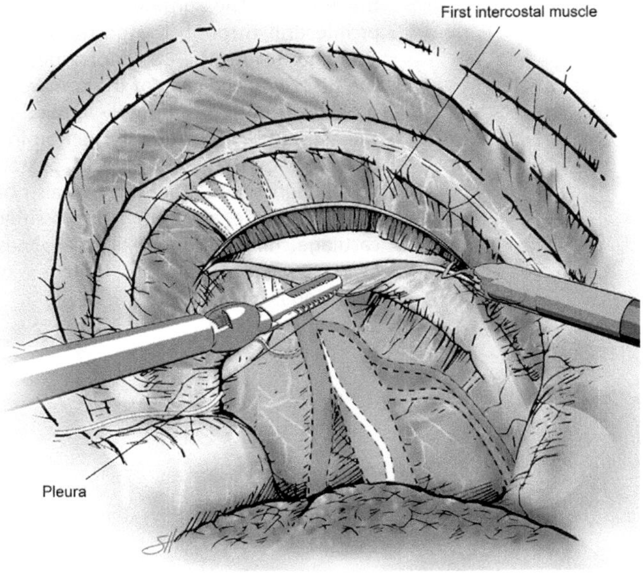


**Fig. 2.** Separation of the first intercostal muscle and dissection of the parietal pleura. The first intercostal muscle is separated from the lateral aspect of the first rib. The pleura is dissected from the underside of the first rib. (Illustration by Scott Holmes. CMI, copyright Baylor College of Medicine.)

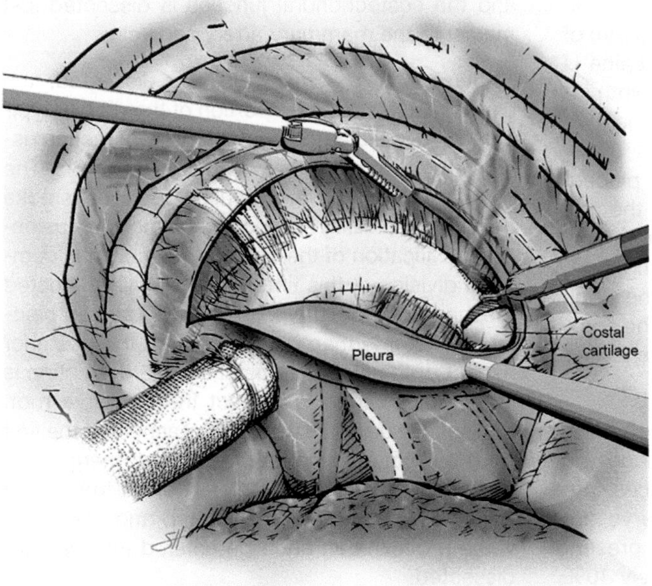


**Fig. 3.** Division of the costal cartilage. The costal cartilage is exposed anteriorly and divided using energy. (Illustration by Scott Holmes. CMI, copyright Baylor College of Medicine.)

process. The drill tip can be used as a tactile probe, and a clear release is usually evident. If the cartilage was ossified and requires division, it can be completed now. The robot is re-docked, and the bipolar dissector is replaced.

***Dissection in the thoracic outlet*** With the rib divided, it can be reflected medially with the Prograsp forceps. The final attachments of the first intercostal muscle as well as the attachments of the serratus anterior muscle are divided with bipolar energy (**Fig. 5**). This further mobilizes the rib and the soft attachments of the superior aspect of the rib to the thoracic outlet can be gently pushed from the rib with a cigar sponge. Coming into view now will be the anterior scalene muscle, the middle scalene muscle (posteriorly), the subclavius muscle (anteriorly), as well as the portions of the subclavian artery, subclavian vein, and the brachial plexus that traverse the thoracic outlet. The neurogenic and venous TOS compression triangles are visualized (**Fig. 6**). Gentle traction is maintained on the first rib to expose these muscles. The attachments of the anterior scalene

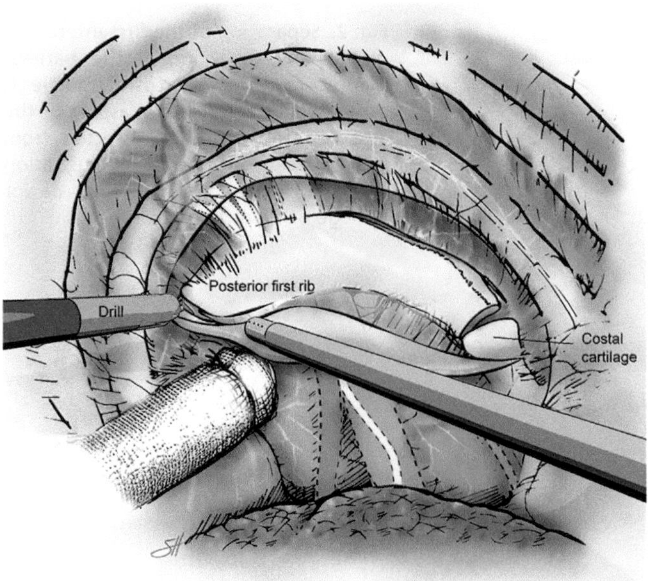


**Fig. 4.** Division of the posterior aspect of the first rib. The surgeon places a low profile drill through the posterior incision and divides the posterior aspect of the first rib at the level of the transverse process. Irrigation is gingerly applied by the assistant by a stationary suction irrigator device that is located to protect the T1 nerve root. The drill can also be used to divide any remaining ossified cartilage. (Illustration by Scott Holmes. CMI, copyright Baylor College of Medicine.)

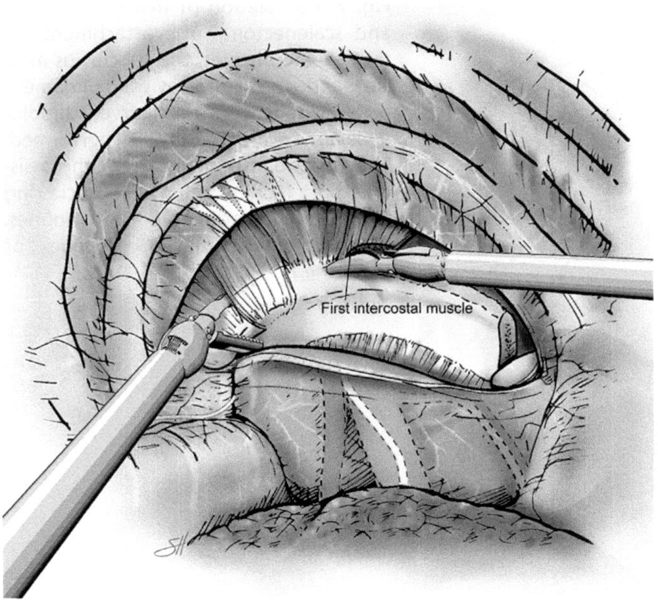


**Fig. 5.** Enter the thoracic outlet. Once the rib is divided anteriorly and posteriorly, the robot is re-docked and the attachments of the remaining first intercostal muscle and the serratus anterior muscle to the first rib are divided. The first rib is reflected medially, and the thoracic outlet is entered. (Illustration by Scott Holmes. CMI, copyright Baylor College of Medicine.)

muscle, middle scalene muscle, subclavius muscle, and costoclavicular ligament are divided precisely where they insert on the first rib (**Fig. 7**). Using the bony rib as a landmark, the surgeon can avoid energy dispersion to adjacent neurovascular structures. The rib is now detached and removed through the assistant port incision with a thoracoscopic grasper.

***Scalenectomy*** The bony compression of the thoracic outlet has now been released, and the surgeon can perform scalenectomy. This is accomplished with gentle grasping of the scalene muscles and a combination of blunt dissection and application of bipolar energy. The extent of scalenectomy is surgeon preference, and we prefer to assure that no muscle is adjacent to neurovascular structures whose compression resulted in symptoms.

***Neurolysis and/or venolysis*** Inflammatory changes and fibrotic tissue are commonly encountered over the subclavian artery/vein and brachial plexus, the degree of which is variable. In patients

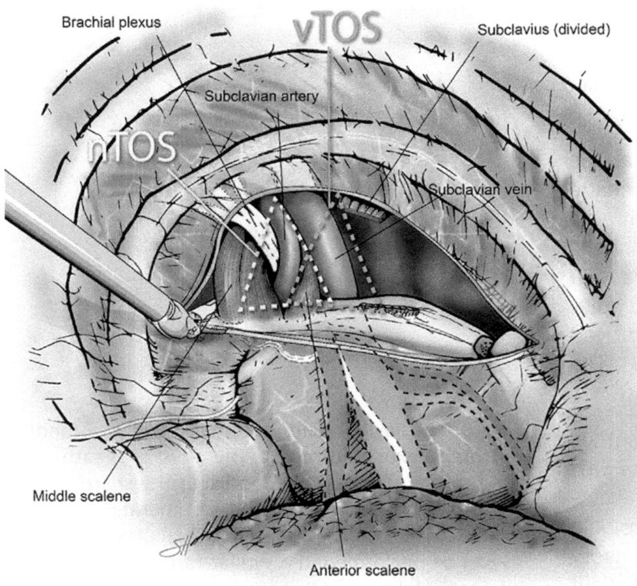


**Fig. 6.** Clarify the anatomy of the thoracic outlet. The borders of the NTOS triangle (middle scalene muscle, first rib, and anterior scalene muscle) and of the VTOS triangle (anterior scalene muscle, first rib, subclavius muscle) are identified. (Illustration by Scott Holmes. CMI, copyright Baylor College of Medicine.)

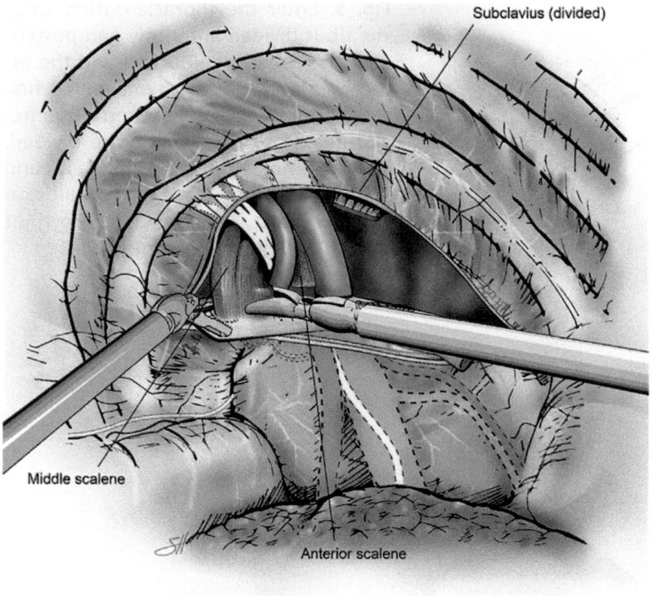


**Fig. 7.** Completion of first rib resection and scalenectomy. The attachments of the scalene muscles, the subclavius muscle, and the costoclavicular ligament are divided with the curved bipolar dissector. Scalenectomy is performed. The first rib is removed from the assistant port incision using a thoracic ring forceps. (Illustration by Scott Holmes. CMI, copyright Baylor College of Medicine.)

with NTOS, it is thought by many that brachial plexus neurolysis can add benefit. Brachial plexus neurolysis can be performed with predominant "sharp" dissection using the relatively pinpoint/sharp tips of the curved bipolar dissector. No energy is typically applied here. The three trunks of the brachial plexus are mobilized from themselves, from the subclavian artery, and from any surrounding fibrotic sheath. Patients with VTOS typically have a more severe extent of fibrosis overlying the subclavian vein and the subclavius muscle and costoclavicular ligament. This fibrosis is dissected in a similar fashion to accomplish a near complete circumferential dissection of the vein where it runs through the thoracic outlet (**Fig. 8**).

***Final intraoperative assessments*** Hemostasis is assured. The reversal of neuromuscular blockade is used for direct visualization of diaphragm contraction, confirming integrity of the phrenic nerve. The robot is de-docked, the camera is reinserted, and 24-French Blake drain is placed adjacent to the thoracic outlet. The ports are removed under direct vision, and the lung is expanded. The port sites are closed in multiple layers.

***Postoperative considerations*** The patient is extubated in the OR at the conclusion of the procedure and is then transferred to the postanesthesia care unit. A thorough focused neurologic examination assessing upper extremity sensory and motor function is performed once the patient has awoken sufficiently from anesthesia. A chest x-ray is obtained. The Blake drain is placed on water seal at midnight and removed the following day. Our analgesia regimen includes preoperative Tylenol and gabapentin, intraoperative rib blocks, standing postoperative Tylenol and gabapentin. Patient-controlled analgesia is used on the day of surgery and transitioned to tramadol as needed on postoperative day 1. Most patients are discharged on the day following surgery.

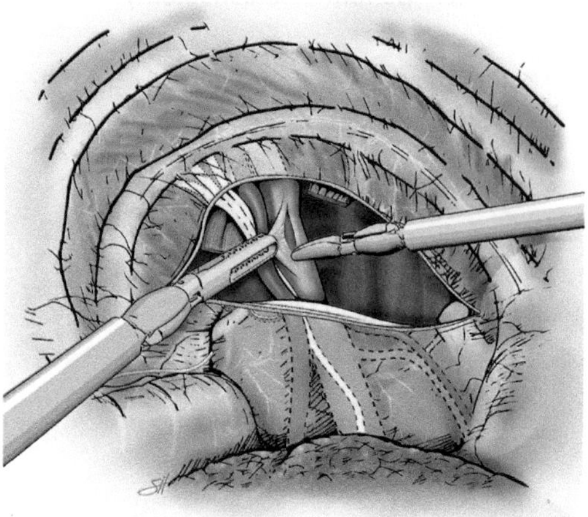

**Fig. 8.** Subclavian vein external venolysis (and/or brachial plexus neurolysis). The fibrous sheath over the brachial plexus is divided using the sharp tips of the curved bipolar dissector to liberate the vein from external compression. A brachial plexus neurolysis can be performed in a similar fashion. (Illustration by Scott Holmes. CMI, copyright Baylor College of Medicine.)

## SUMMARY

Robot-assisted thoracoscopic surgery approaches to first rib resection for TOS are demonstrating good functional outcomes and greatly reduced risk of dreaded neurologic complications. The technique continues to be refined and with greater adoption in the thoracic surgery community. Most institutions with robotic platforms in place have the equipment necessary to perform the operation and the required understanding of thoracic outlet anatomy and technical skills are within the operative armamentarium of most thoracic surgeons.

## CLINICS CARE POINTS

- Robotic first rib resection overcomes the limitations of exposure and risk of manipulation and retraction of neurovascular structures inherent to open first rib resection approaches.
- Thoracic inlet neurovascular structures can clearly be seen before the initiation of dissection and throughout the operation which reduces risk of neurologic complications. An accessory phrenic nerve should be carefully assessed for after port placement.
- Drill activation in pulses allows for precise division while minimizing adjacent heating from the drill bit friction. Intermittent irrigation clears the field and cools the drill.
- Fibrosis around the neurovascular bundle is performed without any cautery to minimize dispersion injury to the structures. Lysis should circumferentially free the neurovascular structures from each other and the adjacent soft tissues.

## DISCLOSURE

Dr B.M. Burt is a proctor and consultant for Intuitive Surgical.

## REFERENCES

1. Christo PJ, McGreevy K. Updated perspectives on neurogenic thoracic outlet syndrome. Curr Pain Headache Rep 2011;15:14–21.
2. Brooke BS, Freischlag JA. Contemporary management of thoracic outlet syndrome. Curr Opin Cardiol 2010;52:406–11.
3. Sanders RJ, Hammond SL, Rao NM. Thoracic outlet syndrome: a review. Neurologist 2008;14:365–73.
4. Burt BM, Palivela N, Cekmecelioglu D, et al. Safety of robotic first rib resection for thoracic outlet syndrome. J Thorac Cardiovasc Surg 2021;162:1297–305.
5. Burt BM, Palivela NP, Karmian A, et al. Transthoracic robotic first rib resection: Twelve steps. JTCVS Tech 2020;1:104–9.

# Three-Dimensional Printing Applications in Thoracic Surgery

Antonia A. Pontiki, BEng[a,b], Kawal Rhode, PhD[a,b], Savvas Lampridis, MD[c], Andrea Bille, MD, PhD[c,d,*]

**KEYWORDS**

• Chest-wall reconstruction • 3D printing • Patient-specific prosthesis • Lobectomy • Simulator • Surgical training

**KEY POINTS**

- Patient-specific chest wall prosthesis was created using 3DP and bespoke computer program.
- Life-size chest simulator was developed for minimally invasive surgical training involving accurate anatomy, high degree of realism, and low cost of production.
- 3D printing can help to plan complex cases to minimize intraoperative complications.

## INTRODUCTION

Three-dimensional (3D) printing (3DP) has been available and used in construction, automotive, and consumer goods since the 1980s.[1] It is an additive manufacturing process that converts a digital model to a physical, 3D object by adding successive layers of material. The first 3DP technique was invented in 1983, by Chuck Hull. Since then, there has been a rapid development of several 3DP techniques all based on the additive manufacturing technique.[2]

The use of 3DP in health care has rapidly increased during the last several years because the technology is readily available, the costs are decreasing,[3] and the reliability of the 3DP products is increasing.[4] Additive manufacturing has also "emerged as an essential technology" during the 2019 COVID-19 pandemic[5] with medical equipment, such as face shields, masks,[6] and valves,[7] being produced rapidly and at low cost, allowing the global health care community to better cope with the supply chain disruption caused by the pandemic. 3DP has shown a great potential because it allows for customized health care solutions but can also be used for prototyping and research. It is progressively used in more medical fields every day to manufacture equipment, develop anatomic models for surgical planning and training, create prostheses, and lately 3D bioprint tissues and organs.[8] Current applications span across many fields of medicine; however, surgical fields have seen the greatest benefit of 3DP. A study including 297 articles from 35 countries showed that 2889 patients benefited from 3D-printed objects, most of them being surgical guides and anatomic models used in dental implant surgery and mandibular reconstruction.[9]

There are no conflicts and/or competing interest.

[a] School of Biomedical Engineering and Imaging Sciences, King's College London; [b] Department of Surgical & Interventional Engineering, School of Biomedical Engineering and Imaging Sciences, The Rayne Institute, St Thomas' Hospital, 4th Floor, Lambeth Wing, London SE1 7EU, UK; [c] Department of Thoracic Surgery, Guy's and St Thomas' NHS Foundation Trust, Guy's Hospital, Great Maze Pond, London SE1 9RT, UK; [d] School of Cancer & Pharmaceutical Sciences, King's College London

* Corresponding author. Department of Thoracic Surgery, Guy's and St Thomas' NHS Foundation Trust, Guy's Hospital, Great Maze Pond, London SE1 9RT, United Kingdom.

*E-mail address:* andrea.bille@gstt.nhs.uk

Twitter: @AntoniaPontiki (A.A.P.); @KawalRhode (K.R.); @SavvasLampridis (S.L.); @AndreaBille (A.B.)

Thorac Surg Clin 33 (2023) 273–281
https://doi.org/10.1016/j.thorsurg.2023.04.012

Surgical education is one of the most significant applications of 3DP, especially for the development of simulation-based training models. Recent studies have reported the use of 3DP in anesthesia to develop a low-cost printed thoracic spine simulator to teach thoracic epidurals to novice anesthesiologists in training programs.[10] Anatomic models are also used presurgically when a complex anatomy is involved in the operation, to plan or simulate the surgery by printing the relevant and complex anatomic structure. An example of that is the use of cardiovascular models for patients with congenital heart disease. Rubber-like 3D-printed heart models allow for preoperative planning and presurgical simulation of the intervention, which can lead to improved outcomes for patients with congenital heart disease.[11] 3DP has also been used to produce a lung, for lung tumor resection and segmentectomy planning.[12,13] The surgical planning using 3D-printed anatomies has led to reduction of unnecessary removal of the lung tissue and hence increased preserved lung capacity. It was also reported that 3D-printed surgical models can reduce operating time, minimize access injury, and prevent air leakage.[13] These advantages make the technology more attractive to surgeons and more commonly used every day.

The use of 3DP has also been very successful in the production of customized, cost-efficient, and readily available implants, especially in the fields of orthopedics, cranial, and maxillofacial surgery.[14] Advances in health care technology allowing the combination of medical imaging and 3DP have greatly benefitted thoracic surgery and have allowed for more complex reconstructions of the chest wall. There have been many cases of 3D-printed titanium chest wall prostheses, including the case completed by Aragon and Mendez,[15] involving the reconstruction of three ribs and the equivalent chondrosternal articulations (**Fig. 1**). The titanium implants were designed based on the patient's computed tomography (CT) images and 3D printed, resulting in an exact replica of the specimen removed from the patient. Wen and colleagues[16] also reported customized titanium-alloy prostheses for the reconstruction of ribs for one patient, and the sternum and bilateral cartilage for another patient. Recently, 3D-printed, custom-made, polyether-ether-ketone (PEEK) implants have been used in China for chest wall reconstruction.[17,18] This method provides patients with the advantage of a perfectly fitted prosthesis, which is directly made from the patients' CT scans. A sternum, 2 to 6 costal cartilage, and ribs prosthesis was created using surgical-grade PEEK and was implanted in combination with a patch (**Fig. 2**). The patient showed no postoperative complications and in follow-up the implant provided enough support to maintain the chest's shape.

## GOALS

Our work explores novel 3DP techniques that, in combination with medical imaging, can be used in thoracic surgery for the creation of patient-specific implants (PSI) and artificial organs, benefitting not only patients, but also clinicians and surgical trainees. The first part of this work uses routine preoperative thoracic CT, acquired as part of a patient with cancer's standard preoperative work-up, and explores the use of 3DP in health care in combination with synthetic materials as a technique to achieve personalized chest wall prostheses for patients undergoing resection surgery as cancer treatment. The personalized rigid prostheses should be able to be implanted with usual surgical techniques, replicate the anatomic structure, restore the functional role of the chest wall, provide protection, and involve a low cost. The ideal product would provide good cosmetic results, and greatly improve a patient's postoperative quality of life, adding further benefits to existing techniques.

The second part focuses on producing a life-size model of the right side of the chest that can be used to simulate video-assisted thoracoscopic surgery (VATS) and robot-assisted thoracoscopic surgery (RATS) lobectomy for surgical training. Current surgical training simulators are not always anatomically accurate and most of them are expensive. The objective was to improve and optimize existing training models, developing a physical, life-size, human chest simulator that is easily reproducible, with a high degree of realism, fidelity, and anatomic accuracy, while maintaining a low manufacturing cost. The chest model should include all anatomic structures involved in a lobectomy and should be compatible with the energy devices used during a VATS/RATS lobectomy, to accurately simulate those surgical procedures.

## APPLICATION

### *Patient-Specific Chest Wall Prostheses Using Three-Dimensional Printing*

Between February 2016 and October 2022, 43 patients underwent chest wall resection and reconstruction for primary or secondary cancer involving the chest wall and were enrolled in the analysis. Twenty-four patients underwent a nonrigid reconstruction using a mesh and 19 patients had a patient-specific 3D rigid reconstruction, based on the methylmethacrylate (MMA) neorib technique described by Suzuki and colleagues.[19] The patient-specific reconstruction started being used

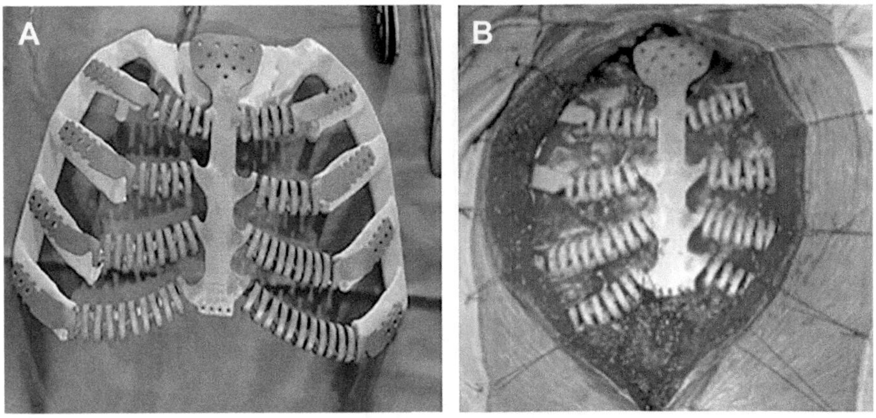

Fig. 1. 3D printed titanium replica of patient's chest wall. (*A*) 3D printed implant. (*B*) Chest wall prosthesis implanted and fixed. (*From* Bustos MEF, España M, Juan S, Sastre I. Sternal reconstruction with 3d titanium prosthesis. Cir Esp (Engl Ed). 2023;101(1):68-70.)

in 2018, so all patients operated before, underwent a mesh nonrigid reconstruction. The 3DP method to produce chest wall PSI models described by Smelt and Pontiki,[20,21] was used to create the prostheses of the patients undergoing chest wall resection and rigid reconstruction for non–small cell lung cancer. The preoperative CT scans of the patients undergoing chest wall resection of two or more ribs were analyzed and the areas of resection were segmented on the CT, as described by Smelt and Pontiki (**Fig. 3**).[20,21] The 3D digital models were then used to produce a 3D print of the chest wall section that was to be resected and reconstructed (**Fig. 4**A), and a silicone mold was created from the 3D-printed model. This mold was sterilized and used to produce MMA prostheses (**Fig. 4**B), which were then implanted into the patients.[20,21]

Since March 2022, an optimized, 3D modeling method that can provide clinicians with a time-efficient technique to create personalized rib prostheses has been used in clinic. The first patient case took place in March 2022 and was reported by Pontiki and colleagues.[22] The novel method described by Pontiki and colleagues[22,23] has been used for two patients since March 2022, who underwent right chest wall resection and reconstruction. To create 3D models of the right ribs three to five for the first patient, and right ribs two to six for the second patient, a bespoke computer program was used that was developed as described by Pontiki and colleagues.[23] The software MATLAB was used, where a program was created to generate rib digital models within seconds. The MATLAB code takes as input the

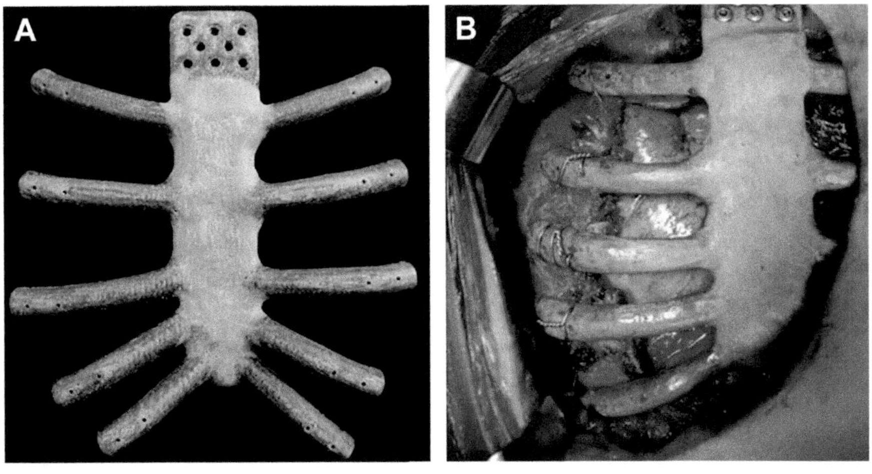

Fig. 2. (*A*) Anterior view of the 3D-printed PEEK sternal prosthesis. (*B*) PEEK prosthesis implanted and fixed on the native ribs using steel wires. (*From* Wang L, Huang L, Li X, et al. Three-Dimensional Printing PEEK Implant: A Novel Choice for the Reconstruction of Chest Wall Defect. Ann Thorac Surg. 2019;107(3):921-928.)

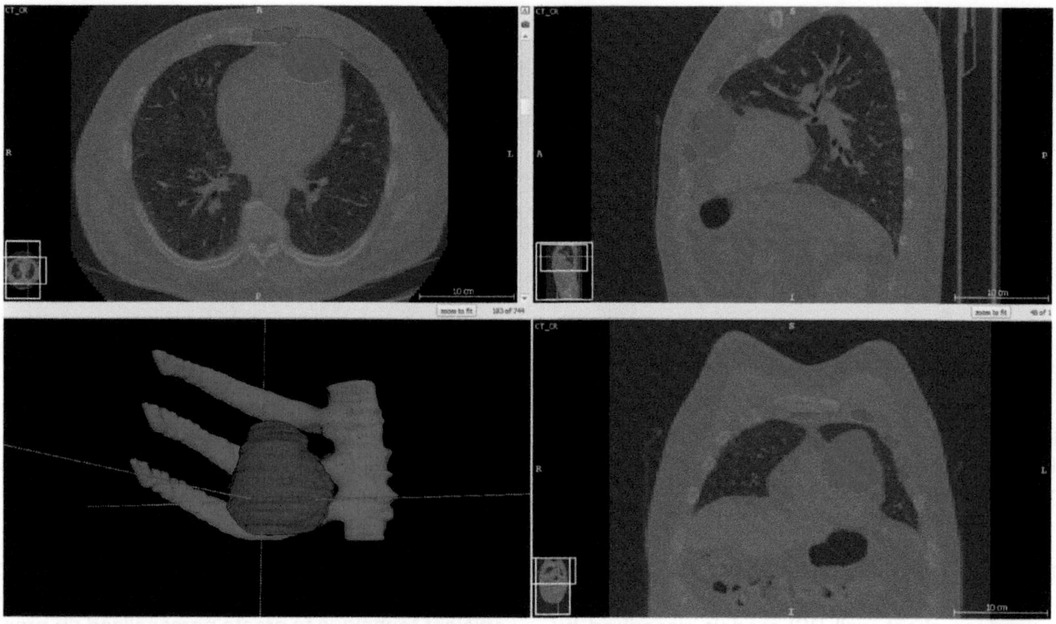

Fig. 3. Preoperative CT segmentation of the sternum and ribs of a patient with chondrosarcoma.

patient's age (years), height (centimeter), weight (kilogram), gender, and the number (2–10) and side (left or right) of ribs. The software generates a digital model for a corresponding rib that would be representative of an "average" patient within this specified demographic. For the two patients, the process was repeated three and five times, respectively, to generate the ribs of interest for each case. The models were generated and processed to keep only the rib segments involved by the tumor, which would then be reconstructed during surgery (**Fig. 5**A). The rib segments were 3D printed in polylactic acid (PLA) filament using the Ender-3 Creality (Shenzhen, China) 3D printer (**Fig. 5**B). The printing of the ribs was completed in approximately 6 hours. The rib prostheses were manufactured in MMA using the silicone mold, following the same method as described previously by Pontiki and colleagues.[20,21]

## *Chest Simulator for Surgical Training*

Minimally invasive thoracic surgery and the use of VATS have gone through fast growth over the past two decades. The rapid advancement in technology and robotics in recent years has also led to a steep increase in the use of RATS. With the rapid evolution of VATS and RATS, there is an increased need for surgical training and improvement of cognitive and procedural skills before operating on patients. The use of surgical simulations has shown promising results in facilitating the training of thoracic surgical trainees because it can provide them with rapid learning in a risk-free and time-efficient manner. Animal models or cadavers are used as an important part of training for thoracic trainee surgeons but involve a high cost and ethical concerns. Virtual reality simulators are used for surgical training but do not provide

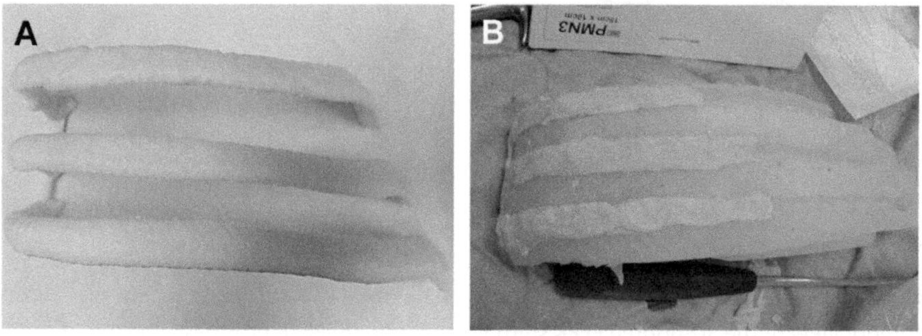

Fig. 4. (*A*) 3D-printed PLA ribs 4, 5, and 6 made by segmenting the CT scan of a patient with lung cancer. (*B*) Silicone mold filled with MMA to make prostheses for the reconstruction of ribs 4, 5, and 6.

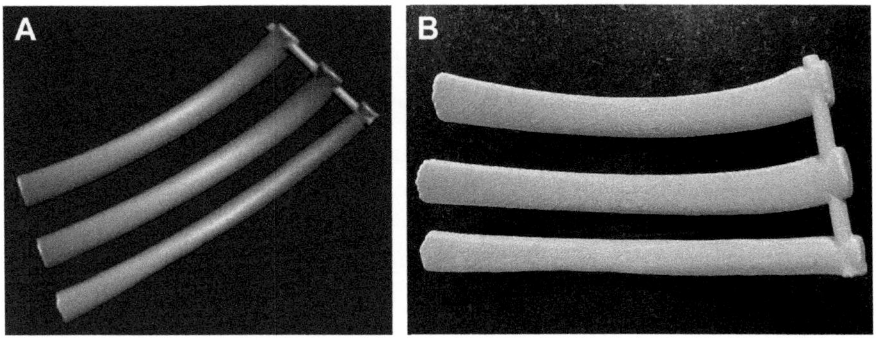


**Fig. 5.** (*A*) 3D digital model of the right 3rd, 4th, and 5th rib sections to be resected and reconstructed. Created using the bespoke computer program. (*B*) 3D-printed right 3rd, 4th, and 5th rib sections in polylactic acid, used to create the silicone mold.

a realistic environment to practice, lacking the feel of texture and tension. Existing artificial physical simulators do not provide an accurate representation of the human anatomy, lacking the different tissue characteristics, blood flow, and electrical conductivity.

A CT scan was used to perform image segmentation as described by Pontiki and colleagues.[21] The segmentation process was carried out to create the structures of interest, which were the anatomies involved in a VATS/RATS lobectomy. Those included the right lung, heart with the aorta, right pulmonary veins and arteries and superior vena cava, trachea and right bronchi (**Fig. 6**), and ribs from the 2nd to the 10th of the right side of the chest wall and right half of the sternum. A base was also designed for the assembly of the simulator, as seen in **Fig. 7**. Three different 3DP techniques and molding were used to manufacture all the anatomic structures of the chest simulator. The heart and pulmonary vessels were 3D printed using the Polyjet 3DP technology[24] with the printer Stratasys Objet Eden 500 and the parts were printed in a soft and flexible rubber called Agilus30 (Stratasys, Eden Prairie, MN). The trachea and bronchi were 3D printed using the Stereolithography 3DP technique,[25] with the Formlabs resin printer Form 3B, in Formlabs Elastic 50A resin (Formlabs, Somerville, MA). The ribcage and base were printed in white PLA (see **Fig. 7**B) using a large Fused Deposition Modeling[26] 3D printer (Chiron, Anycubic, Shenzhen, China). The same printer was used to print the lung mold in PLA filament. That was then used to make the lung in a silicone foam including red pigment for higher realism (SomaFoama15, Smooth-On, Macungie, PA) (see **Fig. 7**A). The previously mentioned materials were chosen based on their mechanical properties, so they could accurately mimic the texture of the respective human tissue.

The novel component of the simulator was the perihilar tissue/mediastinal pleura, which was

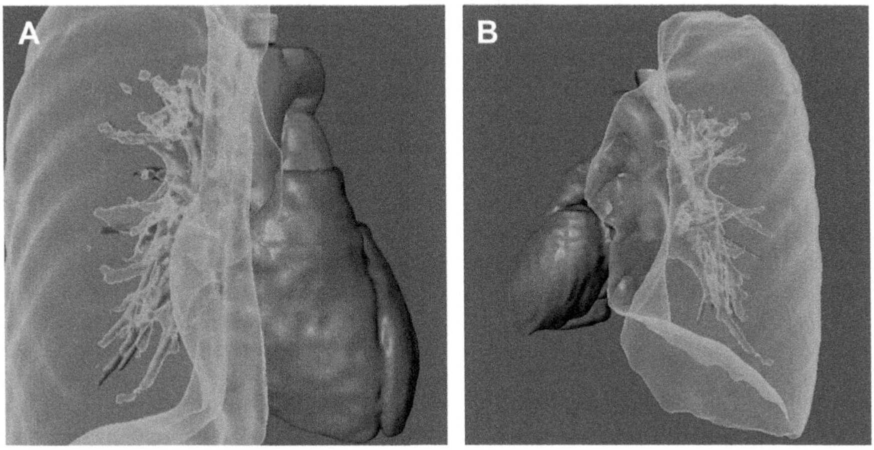


**Fig. 6.** Digital model of the chest simulator. Visualization in Meshmixer of (*A*) close up, anterior view of the heart, vessels, and lung stereolitography (STL) and (*B*) posterior view.

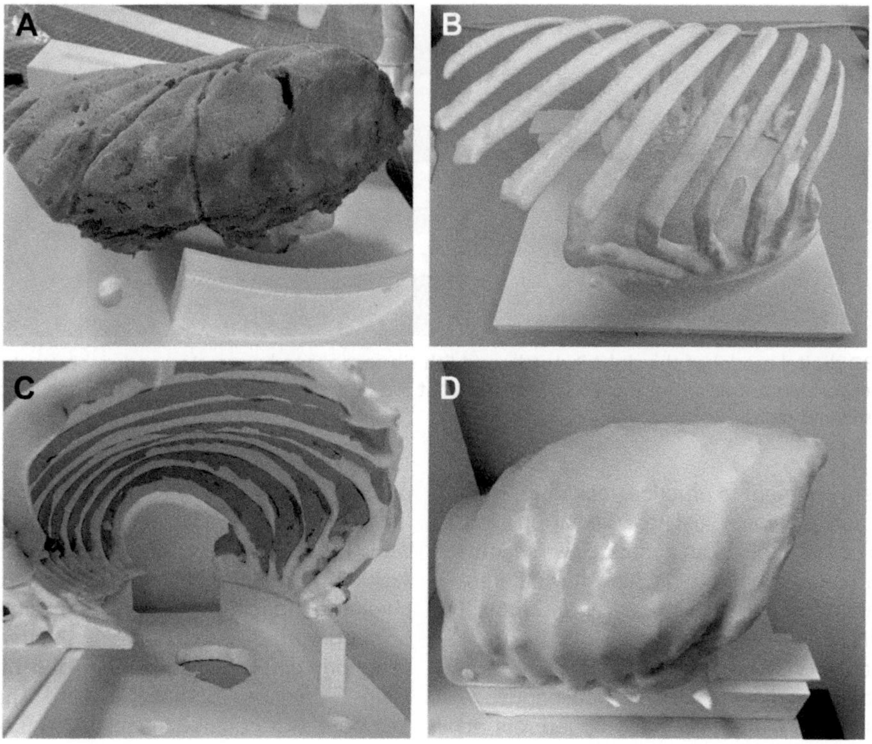


**Fig. 7.** Chest simulator. (*A*) SomaFoama15 lung model attached to the heart and hilum, placed on the 3D-printed base. (*B*) PLA ribcage attached to the base. Agilus30 heart fitted in the heart-shaped hole on the base. (*C*) Inferior view of the ribcage, showing the intercostal muscles made of Brush-On 50. (*D*) Posterior view of the simulator. The ribcage is covered in silicone mimicking the skin.

mimicked by a bespoke material that accurately represented the texture of the tissue, while also being electrically conductive. The material was hydrogel, which made the chest model compatible with energy devices, such as the diathermy and thoracic sealers/dividers. Finally, to further increase the degree of realism of the simulator, the heart model was filled with a blood-mimicking liquid with similar viscosity to blood, to introduce blood flow. This can simulate bleeding when the surgeons cut through the vessels, but it also allows for measuring blood loss during a VATS/RATS lobectomy simulation. The structures were assembled on the 3D-printed base (see **Fig. 7**). A polyurethane rubber compound (Brush-On 50, Smooth-On) was brushed on the ribcage to mimic the intercostal muscles (see **Fig. 7**C), covered with a layer of silicone (EcoFlex0010, Smooth-On) to mimic the skin (see **Fig. 7**D).

## DISCUSSION

Lung cancer is the most common cause of cancer death in the United Kingdom. There are approximately 45,000 new cancer cases per year and the annual cost to the UK economy is an estimated £2.4 b. Lung lobectomy is the most common surgery for lung cancer treatment. Patients with advanced cancer involving the chest wall require en bloc resection surgery and chest wall reconstruction. Lobectomy is the gold standard for early stage lung cancer treatment, with VATS and RATS offering improved surgical outcomes. The use of 3DP for protheses and training models can greatly benefit patients and clinicians in thoracic surgery.

Patient-specific reconstruction of chest wall defects has been completed successfully with the use of 3D-printed titanium-alloy prostheses, as described by Aragon and Mendez[15] and Wen and coworkers,[16] but those are expensive, costing the equivalent of approximately £900 for two ribs,[15,16] compared with our method, which adds £32 to the standard MMA technique. However, Suzuki and coworkers[19] and Pastorino and coworkers[27] have used rigid prostheses of lower cost than titanium, which do not provide a patient-specific reconstruction. The challenge of existing prostheses not being able to provide a low cost and a rigid patient-specific solution was approached using different manufacturing techniques combined. We further developed previously used methods, adding the advantages of using CT scans, 3DP, and silicone molding. Moreover, using the custom MATLAB program to generate the digital rib models provided a less labor-intensive and time-consuming method, which does not require a high level of expertise and any member of the clinical team can create the prostheses.

The use of 3DP in thoracic surgery does not only benefit the patients but can also benefit the clinicians. Currently in thoracic surgery, animals or cadavers are used as an important part of training for surgeons; however, this involves a high-cost and they are subject to quick degradation, so the anatomy is not realistic even after a few hours. Virtual reality simulators are also used for surgical training but do not provide a realistic environment to practice, lacking the feel of texture and tension. Existing artificial physical simulators do not provide an accurate representation of the human anatomy, lacking the different tissue characteristics. The developed model was trialed by thoracic surgeons with encouraging results; the Agilus30 material used for the heart and vessels mimicked well the soft, muscle tissue. The silicone foam lung model was light and flexible for easy retraction and was highly realistic visually and in terms of texture. The intercostal muscles and skin provided a good representation of the chest wall that allows for practicing placing the VATS/RATS ports. Our model is also the first simulator providing electrical conductivity, which mimics the human tissue, so that it can be used with surgical energy devices. The techniques practiced on our model were transferable to a surgical scenario and the use of this model would improve the abilities of a surgical trainee and an experienced surgeon. Moreover, the model allows for repetition of a specific task, without having to complete the entire surgical procedure.

Štupnik and Stork[28] presented a box trainer of high fidelity with a good quality chest wall, which is inexpensive because the endoscopic stapler reloads are revised for infinite use. However, the internal structures lack anatomic accuracy, with the silicone lung inserts being the most significant part of the operation, not presenting a realistic anatomy or texture. The simple tubes representing the blood vessels and bronchi were also inaccurate, not portraying the actual anatomy of the human blood vessels making the simulator not representative of the complete human chest. The commercial model closest to our simulator is that reported by Morikawa and coworkers.[29] The anatomic structures are of high accuracy and quality; however, although the polyvinyl alcohol (PVA) lung and hilum model is also anatomically accurate and has a realistic texture, its disadvantage is the short shelf-life because the lung dries out in a short period of time. This makes the model difficult to transport and store, and in combination with its high cost of production it reduces its accessibility. Our chest simulator addresses all the previously mentioned shortcomings by providing an anatomically accurate model with a high degree of fidelity and realism, while maintaining a low cost of production equal to £500, which is less than 6% of Morikawa's £8700 model[29] and 11% of a cadaver costing near £4500.[30] This model may change the training of not only the new generation of surgeons, but also the theater team to deal with emergency situations, such as acute bleeding or robotic system failure, improving the learning curve with lower costs and higher quality of the models.

## FUTURE DIRECTIONS

### *Chest Wall Reconstruction*

The method for the chest wall prostheses construction described previously is a multistep process, involving intraoperative manufacturing of the implant. A novel 3DP technology to directly print chest wall PSI would save time during surgery by not constructing a new rib on the spot and it would produce a more accurate result than an implant made from a mold. High-performance polymers have shown great potential in cranial, orthopedic, and maxillofacial surgery for the creation of directly 3D-printed prostheses.[31] The key characteristics a biomaterial should possess when being considered for implantation include biocompatibility, sterilizability, and having similar mechanical properties to the human tissue it would replace. Biocompatibility as defined by Williams[32] is "the ability of a material to perform with an appropriate host response in a specific application." The implantable 3D-printed polymer, PEEK, has previously been used to create PSI for surgical reconstructions, such as craniofacial and orthopedic. However, the material has not been used for implantation in the United Kingdom and specifically for thoracic surgical reconstruction. Preliminary mechanical and biocompatibility testing we conducted showed positive results in terms of PEEK's compatibility as a bone replacement material, and implantation for chest wall reconstruction was considered. The existing commercial material VESTAKEEP i4 3DF (Evonik Operations GmbH, Essen, Germany) filament is compliant to ASTM F2026 "Standard Specification for Polyether ether ketone (PEEK) Polymers for Surgical Implant Applications,"[33] and has successfully been used before for implantation. Therefore, a clinical research project will be submitted for ethics approval to the Integrated Research Application System, for the use of PEEK chest wall implants in surgery. Once the research project is approved, a clinical trial will take place at Guy's Hospital to create and implant chest wall prostheses using 3D-printed PEEK. Patients with cancer involving their chest wall, requiring chest wall resection and reconstruction will receive 3D-printed PEEK PSI, and their postoperative outcomes will be recorded and analyzed to assess the material's results.

### *Chest Simulator for Surgical Training*

The physical chest simulator was developed with focus on simulating a right lobectomy; thus, the anatomic structures on the right side (eg, the right lung, right bronchi) were included. However, the model can also be used for training of other procedures. The anatomic structures on the left side of the chest cavity can be included so that a left lobectomy can be simulated. A further procedure that could be simulated on the model is an esophagectomy for esophageal cancer. This is a difficult operation that often involves complications, so a minimally invasive approach is beneficial. VATS and RATS training on the chest simulator can become part of the standard training pathway for thoracic surgical trainees, to provide them with increased surgical exposure before operating on patients.

## SUMMARY

As the technology has become more widely available, the use of 3DP in health care has expanded dramatically. Health care professionals increasingly use 3DP for education, surgical planning and training, and the creation of implantable prostheses. The use of 3DP in this project has demonstrated the unlimited potential this field has to offer. Even though different printing techniques and materials have been used in thoracic surgery, PSI still involves a high cost and a long production period, hence traditional techniques, such as the bone cement sandwich, are still more commonly used. However, 3D-printed anatomic simulators for surgical planning and training are becoming increasingly popular, but they are still highly expensive and without always achieving accuracy and fidelity. The aims are in surgical procedures for thoracic cancer to improve patient outcomes while minimizing the cost of treatment and training of clinicians. The challenge of existing prostheses not being able to provide a low cost and a rigid patient-specific solution was approached in our study with combining different manufacturing techniques. This study further developed previously used methods, adding the advantages of using CT scans, 3DP, and silicone molding to improve the anatomic accuracy of the prosthesis. It was demonstrated that it is possible to create a chest wall PSI that has a solid component (MMA) providing protection, and a flexible component (mesh) that provides compliance.

Finally, a chest surgical simulator was developed and trialed by thoracic surgeons with encouraging results. Limitations of other artificial, surgical simulators include the lack of patient-specific anatomy and of electroconductive characteristics of human tissue. This model is novel and addresses disadvantages of the existing simulators. Based on feedback received, the model is superior to existing ones, offering an anatomically accurate, electrically conductive model with blood flow, and with lower cost compared with cadaveric and animal models. Surgeons need validated tools to practice and improve their skills, especially when the COVID-19 pandemic showed how a training system based on cadavers is not sustainable. This model may change education, patient simulations, and the training of the new generation of surgeons, improving the learning curve with lower costs and higher quality of the models.

## CLINICS CARE POINTS

- Reduced operating time when using the silicone mold to make the MMA prosthesis.
- Reduced cost in providing a patient-specific 3D-printed prosthesis.
- Personalized care for surgical patients.
- Patient-specific simulation model helps to reduce the complications and improve surgical outcome.

## REFERENCES

1. Marro A, Bandukwala T, Mak W. Three-dimensional printing and medical imaging: a review of the methods and applications. Current problems in diagnostic radiology 2016;45(1):2–9.
2. Pechter D. History of 3D Printing – Who Invented the 3D Printer? All3DP. Available at: https://all3dp.com/2/history-of-3d-printing-who-invented-the-3d-printer/. Accessed November 17, 2021.
3. Bhasin V, Bodla MR. Impact of 3D printing on global supply chains by 2020, Massachusetts Institute of Technology 2014. Doctoral Dissertation.
4. Banks J. Adding value in additive manufacturing: researchers in the United Kingdom and Europe look to

3D printing for customization. IEEE pulse 2013;4(6): 22–6.
5. Longhitano GA, Nunes GB, Candido G, et al. The role of 3D printing during COVID-19 pandemic: a review. Progress in Additive Manufacturing 2021;6(1): 19–37.
6. Patric A, Bastawrous S, Bliss J, Burkhardt J. Stopgap Surgical Face Mask (SFM). NIH. Available at: https://3dprint.nih.gov/discover/3dpx-014168. Accessed April 17, 2021.
7. SRL I. Isinnova. Easy Covid. Available at: https://isinnova.it/archivio-progetti/easy-covid-19/. Accessed April 17, 2021.
8. Mashambanhaka F. Medical 3D Printing: The Best Healthcare Applications. All3DP. Available at: https://all3dp.com/2/3d-printing-in-medicine-the-best-applications/. Accessed November 17, 2021.
9. Louvrier A, Marty P, Barrabé A, et al. How useful is 3D printing in maxillofacial surgery? J Stomatol Oral Maxillofac Surg 2017;118(4):206–12.
10. Han M, Portnova AA, Lester M, et al. A do-it-yourself 3D-printed thoracic spine model for anesthesia resident simulation. PLoS One 2020;15(3):e0228665.
11. Lau I, Sun Z. Three-dimensional printing in congenital heart disease: a systematic review. J Med Radiat Sci 2018;65(3):226–36.
12. Kim MP, Ta AH, Ellsworth WA, et al. Three dimensional model for surgical planning in resection of thoracic tumors. Int J Surg Case Rep 2015;16: 127–9.
13. Nakada T, Akiba T, Inagaki T, et al. Thoracoscopic anatomical subsegmentectomy of the right S2b + S3 using a 3D printing model with rapid prototyping. Interact Cardiovasc Thorac Surg 2014;19(4):696–8.
14. Malik HH, Darwood AR, Shaunak S, et al. Three-dimensional printing in surgery: a review of current surgical applications. J Surg Res 2015;199(2): 512–22.
15. Aragón J, Méndez IP. Dynamic 3D printed titanium copy prosthesis: a novel design for large chest wall resection and reconstruction. J Thorac Dis 2016;8(6):E385.
16. Wen X, Gao S, Feng J, et al. Chest-wall reconstruction with a customized titanium-alloy prosthesis fabricated by 3D printing and rapid prototyping. J Cardiothorac Surg 2018;13(1):1–7.
17. Wang L, Liu X, Jiang T, et al. Three-dimensional printed polyether-ether-ketone implant for extensive chest wall reconstruction: a case report. Thorac Cancer 2020;11(9):2709–12.
18. Wang L, Huang L, Li X, et al. Three-dimensional printing PEEK implant: a novel choice for the reconstruction of chest wall defect. Ann Thorac Surg 2019;107(3):921–8.
19. Suzuki K, Park B, Adusumilli PS, et al. Chest wall reconstruction using a methyl methacrylate neo-rib and mesh. Ann Thorac Surg 2015;100:744–7.
20. Smelt J, Pontiki A, Jahangiri M, et al. Three-dimensional printing for chest wall reconstruction in thoracic surgery: building on experience. Thorac Cardiovasc Surg 2020;68(04):352–6.
21. Pontiki AA, Natarajan S, Parker FN, et al. Chest wall reconstruction using 3-dimensional printing: functional and mechanical results. Ann Thorac Surg 2021;S0003-4975(21):01575–7.
22. Pontiki AA, Lampridis S, De Angelis S, et al. Creation of personalised rib prostheses using a statistical shape model and 3D printing: case report. Front Surg 2022;9.
23. Pontiki AA, De Angelis S, Dibblin C, et al. Development and evaluation of a rib statistical shape model for thoracic surgery. In 2022 44th annual International Conference of the IEEE Engineering in medicine & Biology Society (EMBC) 2022 (pp. 3758-3763). IEEE.
24. Gregurić L. What Is Material Jetting? – 3D Printing Simply Explained. All3DP. Available at: https://all3dp.com/2/what-is-material-jetting-3d-printing-simply-explained/. Accessed November 17, 2021.
25. Peltola SM, Melchels FP, Grijpma DW, et al. A review of rapid prototyping techniques for tissue engineering purposes. Ann Med 2008;40(4):268–80.
26. E. National Academies of Sciences and medicine, Predictive Theoretical and Computational Approaches for additive manufacturing: Proceedings of a Workshop. National Academies Press, 2016.
27. Pastorino U, Duranti L, Scanagatta P, et al. Thoraco-pleuropneumonectomy with riblike reconstruction for recurrent thoracic sarcomas. Ann Surg Oncol 2014; 21(5):1610–5.
28. Štupnik T, Stork T. Training of video-assisted thoracoscopic surgery lobectomy: the role of simulators. Shanghai Chest 2018;2:52.
29. Morikawa T, Yamashita M, Odaka M, et al. A step-by-step development of real-size chest model for simulation of thoracoscopic surgery. Interact Cardiovasc Thorac Surg 2017;25(2):173–6.
30. Frick AE, Massard G. Thoracic surgery training in Europe: the perspective of a trainee. J Thorac Dis 2017;9(Suppl 3):S218.
31. Tipton P, Siewert B. High performance polymers part 3. Private Dentistry UK, 2016.
32. Williams DF. On the mechanisms of biocompatibility. Biomaterials 2008;29(20):2941–53.
33. GmbH EO. Product Information VESTAKEEP i4 3DF. Germany: Essen; 2022.

# Uniportal Robotic Lung Resection Techniques

Philicia Moonsamy, MD, MPH[a], Bernard Park, MD[b,*]

**KEYWORDS**

• Minimally invasive surgery (MIS) • VATS • Robotic • RATS • U-VATS (Uniportal VATS)
• U-RATS (Uniportal RATS) • Lung resection

**KEY POINTS**

- Minimally invasive techniques for lung resection are becoming the standard of care.
- Combining a uniportal approach with the technical advantages of telerobotic surgery may afford distinct advantages lacking in multiport video-assisted thoracic surgical (VATS) or robotic-assisted thoracic surgery.
- Clinical experience with uniportal lung resection with multi-arm or single-port robotic systems is in its infancy, but ongoing.

## INTRODUCTION

Telerobotic platforms offer distinct technical enhancements over other minimally invasive surgical (MIS) approaches, including magnified, three-dimensional visualization of the operative field, improved maneuverability of the wristed instruments, ergonomic comfort, and decreased reliance on skilled assistants. Numerous retrospective studies have shown robotic thoracic procedures to be feasible and safe with comparable outcomes to open and video-assisted thoracic surgical (VATS) techniques, and some have even shown improved perioperative outcomes compared to VATS and open, including fewer complications, decreased pain, and need for opioid analgesia and lower 30-day mortality.[1–4] Importantly, robotic approaches have also been shown to achieve equivalent oncologic outcomes for the surgical management of several diseases, such as non-small cell lung cancer (NSCLC)[5] and thymic tumors.[6]

With the accumulation of experience and technological innovation, the utilization of robotics for thoracic surgery has steadily increased since initial Food and Drug Administration (FDA) approval in the late 1990s.[7] During the same period, multiport VATS, defined as utilizing non-rib-spreading incisions less than 8 cm and complete videoscopic dissection, became the most widely accepted MIS approach for advanced pulmonary resections.[8] In 2004, the first series of uniportal VATS (U-VATS) cases was reported for wedge resections and management of benign conditions, such spontaneous pneumothorax.[9] This technique utilizes a single, non-rib-spreading incision less than 8 cm through which all instrumentation is passed. Initially, it was restricted to minor pleural procedures and non-anatomic wedge resection until completion of the first U-VATS lobectomy in 2010 by Gonzalez-Rivas and colleagues.[10] Subsequently, U-VATS has gained popularity in certain regions of the world (Europe, China) with some series showing it to have advantages compared to multiport VATS with respect to chest tube duration and length of stay.[11]

There are many theoretical pros and cons to each of the MIS techniques and, unfortunately, for many reasons, not the least of which is lack of clinical equipoise, there are few prospective, controlled trials with which to compare them; however, with a plethora of retrospective outcome

[a] Division of Thoracic Surgery, Massachusetts General Hospital, 55 Fruit Street, Austen 7, Boston, MA 02114, USA; [b] Thoracic Service, Memorial Sloan-Kettering Cancer Center, 1275 York Avenue, Room C-879, New York, NY 10065, USA
* Corresponding author.
*E-mail address:* parkb@mskcc.org

Thorac Surg Clin 33 (2023) 283–289
https://doi.org/10.1016/j.thorsurg.2023.04.006

data, there are several conclusions about MIS for lung resections that are well-established.[11,12] First, compared with open thoracotomy MIS is associated with decreased chest tube duration, shorter length of stay, and fewer complications. Second, use of MIS for the primary treatment of lung cancer is oncologically acceptable. Third, in terms of perioperative outcomes, robotic and VATS approaches are similar. Detractors of the multiport robotic approach cite cons that include the initial learning curve, increased costs, and variable access to the technology. Although some studies have shown that use of the multiport robotic system is associated with increased in-hospital charges,[13] others have shown that much of these charges are offset by decreased post-operative costs associated with shorter length of stay and decreased complication rate.[14,15] Thus, patients will likely continue to prefer smaller and fewer incisions if surgeons can continue to offer this with no compromise in oncologic outcomes.

Because of increasing utilization of MIS and differences in robotic and non-robotic techniques, there has been recent interest in converging the fields of uniportal surgery and robotics to combine the advantages of the two. This has been further stimulated by the advancement of the first single-port (da Vinci SP) platform developed in 2018 by Intuitive Surgical (Sunnyvale, California, USA). Here, we review the existing published experience with uniportal robotic-assisted thoracic surgery (U-RATS), outlining the techniques utilizing the traditional multi-arm versus the new SP platform.

## UNIPORTAL ROBOTIC-ASSISTED THORACIC SURGERY: MULTI-ARM PLATFORM

The original and subsequent generations of the telerobotic surgery platforms employ a multi-arm surgical cart, and complex thoracic procedures are traditionally performed through a multiple incision (3 or 4) strategy (one incision for each arm). There have been recent reports of U-RATS in the literature utilizing the multi-arm platform through a single incision without rib spreading.[16–18] In 2021, Yang and colleagues[16] reported a case of a right upper lobe lobectomy performed by a hybrid U-RATS approach using the da Vinci Xi system. With the patient placed in a left lateral decubitus position, the authors created a 4 cm incision in the fourth intercostal space in the mid-axillary line, and the surgical cart is "moved to the cranial side and slightly turned to the back" parallel to the patient's rib spaces. Only three of the robotic arms were used with the 30° scope placed in the most posterior (upper) aspect of the incision with the other two working ports placed anteriorly to the camera. The bedside assistant provided additional support through the anterior portion of the incision. Of note, in their approach, the two working arms were crossed inside the chest requiring control to be reset on the surgeon's console. The robotic instruments (Cadiere and hook monopolar cautery) were used to perform hilar dissection; however, ultimately the bedside assistant isolated and stapled the vascular and bronchial structures with non-robotic instrumentation (clamp and handheld staplers). The authors performed a standard anterior-to-posterior approach to the right upper lobectomy which was accomplished in approximately 90 minutes. The patient was discharged on post-operative day 3 without complication.

In the same year, Gonzalez-Rivas and colleagues described a similar technique for U-RATS in performing a left lower lobe lobectomy and a right upper lobe segmentectomy via a single 3 to 5 cm intercostal incision in the fifth intercostal space without rib spreading.[17] The major difference between their approach and the previous report by Yang was that they recommended a "pure" robotic procedure using only robotic instrumentation for dissection and ligation of all structures. Once again, three arms were used to avoid collisions with the camera arm placed in the most posterior aspect of the incision and the working arms were placed adjacently in parallel so that they did not cross (**Fig. 1**). The authors preferred two bipolar instruments (Maryland and fenestrated forceps) for dissection, and the bedside assistant accessed the incision through the most anterior aspect for suction and retraction. The robotic stapler was utilized for ligation of the hilar structures and fissures. The advantages proposed for U-RATS were potentially quicker (compared with multiportal robotics) emergent conversion and greater facility in achieving "complex resections."

More recently, Vincenzi and colleagues[18] reported two cases using the daVinci Xi system for U-RATS in the surgical treatment of early-stage NSCLC. The technique described was essentially identical to that suggested by Gonzalez-Rivas and colleagues. with only minor variations in the interspace used (sixth), as well as utilization of a wound retractor and, similarly to the report by Yang and colleagues, a hybrid technique was used whereby ligation of the hilar structures was performed by the bedside assistant using handheld clip appliers and staplers. The two cases were a left lower lobe superior segmentectomy (S6) and a right lower lobectomy. Neither patient suffered any post-operative complications and length of stay was 5 and 4 days, respectively.

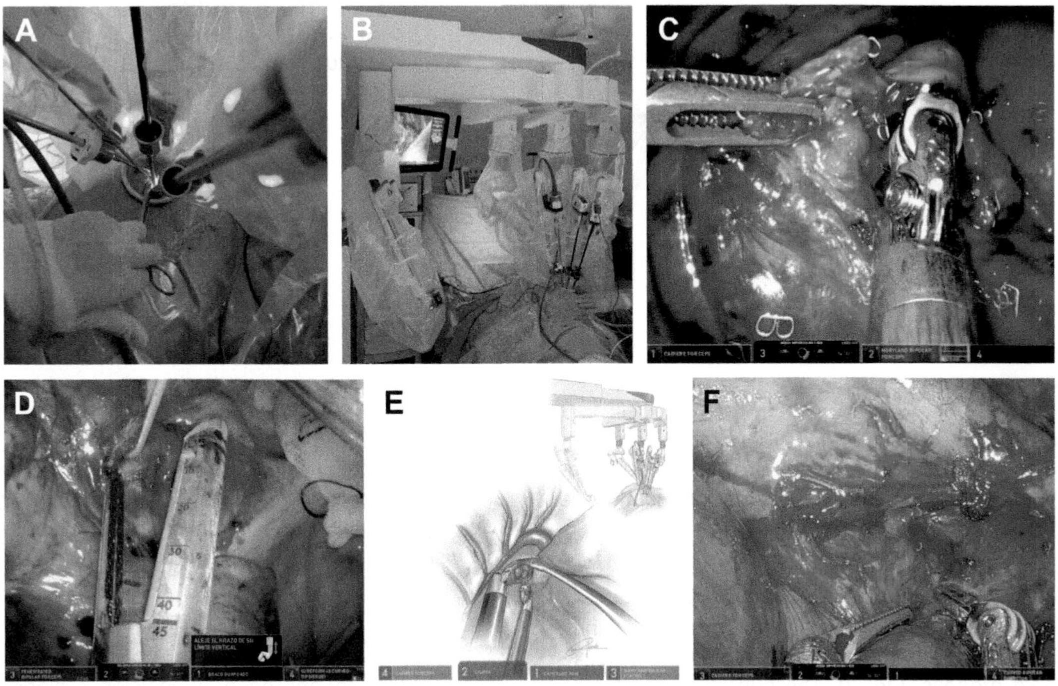

**Fig. 1.** (*A*) Robotic arms configuration (as U-VATS): posterior arm with port—camera, middle, and anterior arms; (*B*) all three arms joints parallel at the top and centered in FLEX position, all rotated toward anterior; (*C*) dissection: Maryland Bipolar Forceps, Cadiere Forceps; (*D*) exposure with short-vessel loop; (*E*) lymph-node-dissection exposure with assistant handling the suction; (*F*) energy grasping instruments in both hands allows swapping configurationleft-right (eg, subcarinal). (*From* Gonzalez-Rivas D, Bosinceanu M, Motas N, Manolache V. Uniportal robotic-assisted thoracic surgery for lung resections. Eur J Cardiothorac Surg. 2022;62(3):ezac410.)

Overall, the key takeaways from this report were that combining the benefits of the uniportal approach including shorter length of stay and shorter chest tube duration with the improved three-dimensional visualization and maneuverability of the robotic platform can be advantageous.

These reports begin to suggest that anatomic resection including segmentectomy is feasible and safe through the uniportal approach using the Xi platform. However, the authors do report that the lack of triangulation and narrow operating field through the uniportal incision caused multiple collisions with the robotic instruments and made this approach more demanding than the multiportal robotic approach. Utilizing the Xi platform for a uniportal approach therefore undoubtedly requires previous training and comfort with U-VATS techniques to achieve acceptable operative times and successful outcomes.

## UNIPORTAL ROBOTIC-ASSISTED THORACIC SURGERY: SINGLE-PORT PLATFORM

The only commercially available single-port telerobotic platform (da Vinci SP) was developed in 2018 by Intuitive Surgical (Sunnyvale, California, USA) and has been FDA-approved for urological procedures and TransOral Robotic Surgery (TORS) for head and neck operations. It is not currently approved for thoracic indications in the United States. The SP platform consists of a single 2.5 cm cannula with four working channels through which three multi-jointed Endowrist instruments and the three-dimensional high-definition articulating endoscope are passed (**Fig. 2**). The instruments are interchangeable and can be placed into different configurations throughout the operation. The robotic arms have seven degrees of freedom which allows range of motion in the chest beyond what can be achieved with both VATS and open approaches. As with the multiport platform, the surgeon sits at a free-standing console and manipulates the instruments with two master controls, one for each hand. The motions of the surgeon's hand can be scaled down by robotic technology, which allows elimination of physiologic tremor.

Given concerns that the 2.5 cm uniportal cannula may not reliably fit through the rib spaces of all patients, the development of da Vinci SP techniques for thoracic indications has focused on a

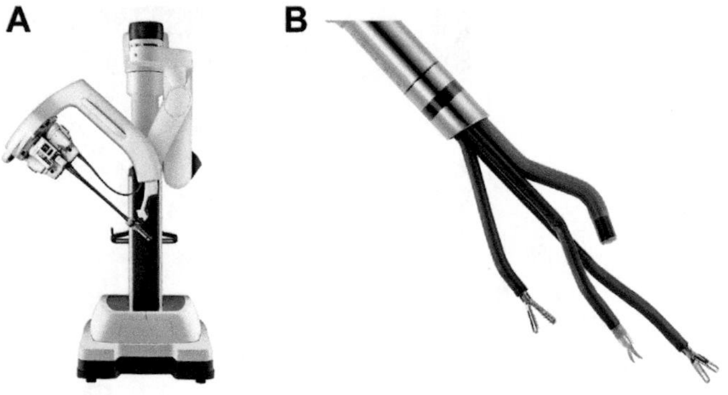

**Fig. 2.** The da Vinci SP system. (*A*) Surgical cart; (*B*) Cannula with instruments. (© 2023 Intuitive Surgical Operations, Inc.)

subxiphoid or subcostal approach. Gonzalaz-Rivas was instrumental in the pre-clinical development of a technical strategy for implementing da Vinci SP for thoracic procedures.[19]

## Subxiphoid Approach

For the subxiphoid approach, a 4 cm vertical incision is made just over the prominence of the xiphoid process (**Fig. 3**). The subcutaneous tissue is opened, and the rectus muscles are incised near the insertions to the costal arches at the midline. The cartilaginous xiphoid process is excised using scissors. The anterior mediastinum is opened from below the sternum, and a retrosternal tunnel is created by blunt finger dissection to open the pleural cavity. One should avoid violating the diaphragm to prevent the risk of a future diaphragmatic hernia. An access gel port is placed (GelPOINT, Applied Medical Corporation, Rancho Santa Margarita, California, USA) through which the 2.5 cm SP robotic trocar is placed. The GelPOINT access port allows $CO_2$ insufflation to 8 to 10 mm Hg, a must to increase the space and visibility in the chest, particularly on the left side.

## Subcostal Approach

For the subcostal approach, an incision is placed lateral to the xiphoid process approximately 1 cm and is parallel to the subcostal margin (**Fig. 3**). Following division of the rectus abdominus fibers, the plane just beneath the costal margin is developed bluntly and the chest is entered digitally. The GelPOINT access gel port is placed and $CO_2$ insufflation is initiated. The 2.5 cm SP robotic trocar is docked, and an additional 12 mm trocar is inserted through the GelPOINT device side by side to the SP robotic trocar for the

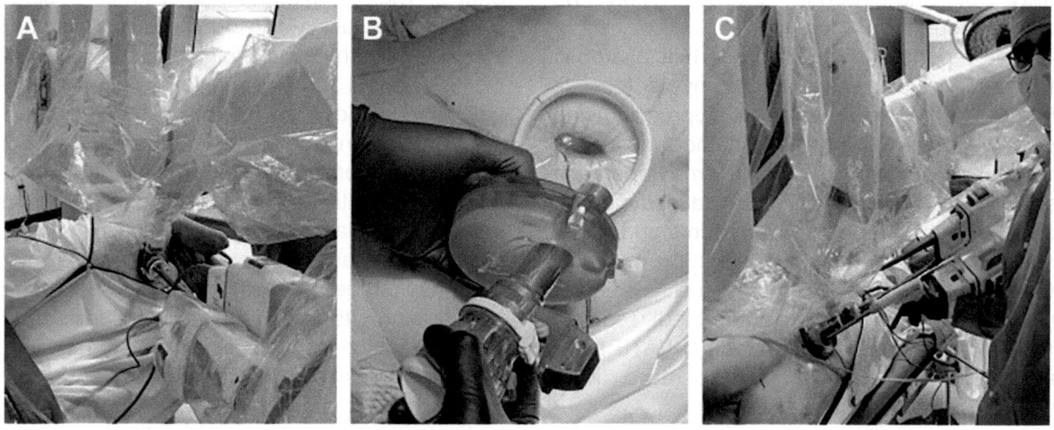

**Fig. 3.** Position for subxiphoid and subcostal approach. (*A*) Lateral decubitus position, subxiphoid incision with GelPOINT system adapted and 2.5 cm trocar showing the four working channels; (*B*) right subcostal incision and direction of GelPOINT system to be adapted to the wound protector (the additional thoracic incision is made to control from inside movements of the robot during experimental surgery); (*C*) stapler insertion by the surgeon during a left upper lobectomy. (*From* Gonzalez-Rivas D, Ismail M. Subxiphoid or subcostal uniportal robotic-assisted surgery: early experimental experience. J Thorac Dis. 2019;11(1):231-239.)

assistant to insert staplers, for suctioning, or to facilitate lung retraction and exposure if needed.

### Hilar and Mediastinal Dissection

Once the SP surgical cart is docked, dissection can be performed according to each surgeon's preference depending on the specific type of anatomic resection planned and the patient's individual condition. Ligation of the hilar structures was performed either by application of robotic clips or staplers passed by the bedside assistance through the gelport. Gonzalez-Rivas noted several pros and cons of the SP approach compared to a VATS subxiphoid/subcostal alternative. The advantages included enhanced ergonomic exposure and dissection, improved triangulation of the instruments, superior view, mitigation of physiologic tremor, and ease of performance of systematic lymph node dissection. Among the disadvantages of the robotic approach were the theoretical cost, learning curve, lack of robotic stapling and reliance, therefore, on the bedside assistant, lack of haptic feedback as well as potential for emergency conversion without the operating surgeon being at the bedside.

### Current Status of da Vinci Single-Port Anatomic Lung Resection

Based on the initial pre-clinical work done by Gonzalez-Rivas, a follow-up pre-clinical study of the da Vinci SP system was conducted by Wu and colleagues[20] designating a subxiphoid approach for thymectomy and a subcostal strategy for lobectomy in three cadaver models (**Fig. 4**). Four subcostal anatomical lung resections and two subxiphoid thymectomies were completed without requiring additional incisions. In this study, a new access kit was introduced for the 4 cm subcostal incision, the da Vinci SP Access Port Kit through which the 2.5 cm SP trocar is inserted, and which allows for bedside assistance and stapling. The refinements achieved in this follow-up study provided the basis for the ensuing clinical trial of the system for thoracic surgical indications. A multicenter, prospective Investigational Device Exemption trial of the use of the da Vinci SP Surgical System for thymectomy and lobectomy is now underway in the United States. The trial began enrolling in July 2022 with the primary completion date estimated to be sometime in December 2023 (https://clinicaltrials.gov/ct2/show/NCT05150210?cond=da+vinci+sp&draw=2). The primary endpoint will be safety with a variety of secondary endpoints, including perioperative outcomes and 5-year oncologic outcomes.

## SUMMARY

MIS approaches (VATS and robotic) for anatomic lung resection are becoming the standard of care because of well-established benefits to the patient that include decreased surgical trauma afforded by avoidance of prolonged rib spreading and soft tissue injury, decreased rate and severity of postoperative complications, shorter length of hospital stay, enhanced recovery, and oncologic equivalence. Technological advances and growing clinical experience have resulted in ongoing innovation that has led to widespread adoption and expansion of the indications and complexity of the cases such that there are few that cannot be considered for MIS.

In the case of VATS, the progression of the approach in the last 25 years has been from establishing a stnadrad definition to demonstrating efficacy and expanding its adoption to include locally advanced disease all while reducing the required number of incisions to one (uniportal). The emergence of telerobotic technology added immediate enhancements for the MIS surgeon: binocular vision with re-establishment of depth perception, wristed instrumentation with tremor control and ergonomic comfort, but with increased costs, loss of tactile feedback, and unclear patient benefits. Innovations in robotic technology that simplified implementation and introduced advanced instrumentation (stapling) have stimulated expanding adoption and greater experience has suggested patient benefits as well.

Yet, neither VATS nor robotic approaches are in themselves perfect, and so it seems that an effort to merge the very best elements of each seems logical and inevitable. U-RATS is an attempt to combine the simplicity of employing a single incision with the enhanced vision and instrumentation of telerobotic systems, whether it is with a multiport or SP system. This strategy makes several assumptions that are not necessarily valid.

1. *One incision is better than multiple small ones.* There have been several efforts to show a difference between uniportal and multiport VATS in the treatment of primary lung cancer, and the results have been mixed. Perhaps the greatest potential difference would be in postoperative pain; however, while this has been suggested by the practitioners of U- VATS, it has never been proven in a rigorous fashion.
2. *U-RATS will be equally safe and oncologically efficacious.* Although there are initial reports of the feasibility of U-RATS with the da Vinci Xi system, they have either been from the recognized authority on complex U-VATS[17] or utilizing a

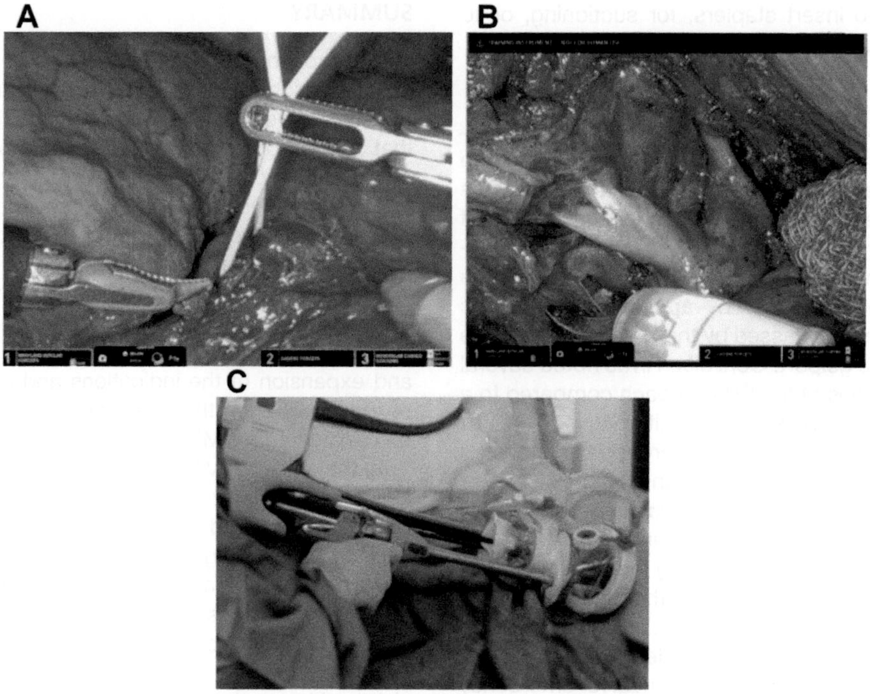

**Fig. 4.** The target pulmonary artery was encircled with a vessel loop. (*A*) Expansion of the working space to allow safe entering of the staple was achieved through (*B*) an extensive dissection along the pulmonary vessels. (*C*) The stapler was introduced through the assistant port of the da Vinci SP Access Port Kit via a subcostal incision. (*From* Wu CF, Cheng C, Suen KH, Stein H, Chao YK. A Preclinical Feasibility Study of Single-Port Robotic Subcostal Anatomical Lung Resection and Subxiphoid Thymectomy Using the da Vinci® SP System. Diagnostics (Basel). 2023;13(3):460. Published 2023 Jan 26)

hybrid technique[18] that is not a "pure" robotic procedure. Having a single incision positioned outside the thorax proper and a distance away from the hilar anatomy may make management of vascular emergencies a challenge.

3. *Costs will be similar.* Cost comparisons of telerobotic surgery with non-robotic MIS are challenging, particularly if not performed prospectively and require complex financial models that account for multiple factors, including, but not limited to, amortization schedules, depreciation, and inflation. Add to this that the SP system is relatively new with few approved indications, and it will be difficult to assess the cost of adoption relative to U-VATS or multiport robotic cases.
4. *U-RATS will provide technical benefits for surgeons.* For U-VATS surgeons, they must contend with the learning curve associated with telerobotic surgery (docking, instrument collisions, loss of tactile sensation, reliance on visual feedback) and a fundamentally different dissection methodology. Multiport VATS surgeons must contend with all of this and adjusting to working through a single incision. Similarly, multiport robotic surgeons will need to adapt to a new telerobotic platform that has different performance characteristics (instrument movement, lack of robotic stapling), as well as a completely foreign incision strategy.

Ultimately, U-RATS (employing the da Vinci Xi or SP platform) for anatomic lung resection will need to be feasible, and the effort to demonstrate this is ongoing through individual efforts and a multicenter prospective trial. Assuming either or both strategies prove to be so, the challenge for the manufacturer and early adopters will be to work together to design subsequent prospective, controlled trials which define the optimal role in the surgical management of lung cancer and other thoracic diseases.

## CLINICS CARE POINTS

- Currently the only option for uniportal robotic lung resection outside of the ongoing clinical trial is to utilize the multiport system through a single incision
- Uniportal robotic lung resection requires a highly skilled bedside assistant

- Initial cases of uniportal robotic cases should be limited to localized lesions in good risk patients

## FUNDING

This work was supported, in part, by National Institutes of Health/National Cancer Institute [Cancer Center Support Grant P30 CA008748].

## DISCLOSURE

Dr P. Moonsamy has no disclosures; Dr B. Park has received honoraria from Intuitive Surgical.

## REFERENCES


1. Park BJ, Flores RM, Rusch VW. Robotic assistance for video-assisted thoracic surgical lobectomy: technique and initial results. J Thorac Cardiovasc Surg 2006;131:54–9.
2. Cerfolio RJ, Bryant AS, Skylizard L, et al. Initial consecutive experience of completely portal robotic pulmonary resection with 4 arms. J Thorac Cardiovasc Surg 2011;142:740–6.
3. Dylewski MR, Ohaeto AC, Pereira JF. Pulmonary resection using a total endoscopic robotic video-assisted approach. Semin Thorac Cardiovasc Surg 2011;23:36–42.
4. Park BJ, Melfi F, Mussi A, et al. Robotic lobectomy for non-small cell lung cancer (NSCLC): long-term oncologic results. J Thorac Cardiovasc Surg 2012;143:383–9.
5. Farivar AS, Cerfolio RJ, Vallieres E, et al. Comparing robotic lung resection with thoracotomy and video-assisted thoracoscopic surgery cases entered into the Society of Thoracic Surgeons database. Innovations 2014;9:10–5.
6. Marulli G, Maessen J, Melfi F, et al. Multi-institutional European experience of robotic thymectomy for thymoma. Ann Cardiothorac Surg 2016;5:18–25.
7. Alwatari Y, Khoraki J, Wolfe LG, et al. Trends of utilization and perioperative outcomes of robotic and video-assisted thoracoscopic surgery in patients with lung cancer undergoing minimally invasive resection in the United States. JTCVS Open 2022;12:385–8.
8. Swanson SJ, Herndon JE 2ND, D'Amico TA, et al. Video-assisted thoracic surgery lobectomy: report of CALGB 39802–a prospective, multi-institution feasibility study. J Clin Oncol 2007;25:4993–7.
9. Rocco G, Martin-Ucar A, Passera E. Uniportal VATS wedge pulmonary resections. Ann Thorac Surg 2004;77:726–8.
10. Gonzalez D, Paradela M, Garcia J, et al. Single-port video-assisted thoracoscopic lobectomy. Interact Cardiovasc Thorac Surg 2011;12:514–5.
11. Magouliotis DE, Fergadi MP, Spiliopoulos K, et al. Uniportal versus multiportal video-Assisted thoracoscopic lobectomy for Lung Cancer: an updated meta-analysis. Lung 2021;199:43–53.
12. Mattioni G, Palleschi A, Mendogni P, et al. Approaches and outcomes of Robotic-Assisted Thoracic Surgery (RATS) for lung cancer: a narrative review. J Robotic Surg 2022. https://doi.org/10.1007/s11701-022-01512-8.
13. Swanson SJ, Miller DJ, McKenna RJ Jr, et al. Comparing robot assisted thoracic surgical lobectomy with conventional video-assisted thoracic surgical lobectomy and wedge resection: results from a multihospital database (Premier). J Thorac Cardiovasc Surg 2014;157:929–37.
14. Kneuertz PF, Singer E, D'Souza DM, et al. Hospital cost and clinical effectiveness of robotic-assisted versus video-assisted thoracoscopic and open lobectomy: A propensity score-weighted comparison. J Thorac Cardiovasc Surg 2019;157:2018–26.
15. Nasir BS, Bryant AS, Minnich DJ, et al. Performing robotic lobectomy and segmentectomy: cost, profitability, and outcomes. Ann Thorac Surg 2014;98:203–8.
16. Yang Y, Song L, Huang J, et al. A uniportal right upper lobectomy by three-arm robotic-assisted thoracoscopic surgery using the da Vinci (Xi) Surgical System in the treatment of early-stage lung cancer. Transl Lung Cancer Res 2021;10:1571–5.
17. Gonzalez-Rivas D, Bosinceanu M, Motas N, et al. Uniportal robotic-assisted thoracic surgery for lung resections. Eur J Cardio Thorac Surg 2022;62. https://doi.org/10.1093/ejcts/ezac410.
18. Vincenzi P, Lo Faso F, Eugeni E, et al. Uniportal robotic-assisted thoracoscopic surgery for early-stage lung cancer with the Da Vinci Xi: Initial experience of two cases. Int J Med Robot 2023;19:e2477. https://doi.org/10.1002/rcs.2477.
19. Gonzalez-Rivas D, Ismail M. Subxiphoid or subcostal uniportal robotic-assisted surgery: early experimental experience. J Thorac Dis 2019;11:231–9.
20. Wu CF, Cheng C, Suen KH, et al. A preclinical feasibility study of single-port robotic subcostal anatomical lung resection and subxiphoid thymectomy using the da Vinci® SP System. Diagnostics 2023;13:460.

# Lung Xenotransplantation

Anthony M. Swatek, MD, Kalpaj R. Parekh, MBBS*

**KEYWORDS**

• Thoracic surgery • Lung transplantation • Lung xenotransplantation • Xenograft

**KEY POINTS**

- A shortage of donor lungs suitable for transplantation is resulting in deaths of patients who have end-stage lung disease and are on the waiting list.
- One means of expanding the number of donor lung allografts is lung xenotransplantation.
- Clinical application of lung xenotransplantation is not possible currently due to xenograft rejection.
- Lung xenotransplantation into humans is on the horizon because of recent advances in the areas of cellular biology, molecular biology, and tissue engineering.
- Remaining concerns with lung xenotransplantation relate to infectious complications and ethical considerations.

## BACKGROUND

Lung transplantation remains the definitive treatment for a variety of pulmonary pathologies when nonsurgical therapies fail. However, for a variety of reasons, transplantation of human lung allografts is not always possible. A key problem is that the supply of organ donors available for transplantation is inadequate. A second issue is that when organ donors become available, their lung utilization for transplantation is only approximately 20%.[1] Often, by the time a donor lung becomes available, the transplant recipient has become too sick to benefit from the surgery or has died (in 2020, this was the case for 15% of lung transplant candidates on waitlist in North America).[1,2] The fact that the lung allograft donor pool is insufficient to meet the growing need for viable organs has stimulated research on lung xenotransplantation, that is, the transplantation of a lung from another species. Although xenotransplantation of the lung has lagged behind attempts at xenotransplantation of other solid organs, recent advances in the ability to rapidly alter the genetics of xenograft donors represent an exciting new opportunity for progress in the field.

Although outcomes from organ allotransplantation continue to improve, and other efforts have been made to increase the donor organ supply, hundreds of people continue to die on the waiting list.[3] Xenotransplantation is a potentially unlimited source of organs that could be delivered in a timely and well-controlled clinical scenario. The potential for, and perceived benefits of, xenotransplantation into humans were recognized long ago, with the perfusion of humans with blood from several species having been reported as early as the 17th century. Since then, frog skin, chimpanzee testis, chimpanzee kidney, chimpanzee heart, chimpanzee liver, and pig islets have been transplanted into humans. Most notably, a pig-to-human heart transplant was performed in January 2022.[3–5]

The pig heart to human xenotransplant, which was performed at the University of Maryland, USA, has brought xenotransplantation to the forefront as a potential solution to the organ shortage, which applies to other organs as well as the lung. Notably, although attempts have been made to transplant various organs, including heart, from multiple species into humans, no clinical reports of lung xenotransplantation into human recipients are available.[6]

Department of Cardiothoracic Surgery, University of Iowa Hospitals and Clinics, 200 Hawkins Drive, SE500GH, Iowa City, IA 52242, USA
* Corresponding author.
*E-mail address:* kalpaj-parekh@uiowa.edu

Thorac Surg Clin 33 (2023) 291–297
https://doi.org/10.1016/j.thorsurg.2023.04.010
1547-4127/23/

There have, however, been significant contributions from multiple investigators studying xenotransplantation, in general, including those of renowned surgeon-scientist David K.C. Cooper, MD, who has recently returned to the Harvard University programs, as well as, Burcin Esker, MD, PhD, out of the University of Indiana. Special mention should be made regarding the significant research and writing contributions specifically regarding lung xenotransplantation, including those of Richard N. Pierson III, MD, working closely with Lars Burdorf, MD, both recently at the University of Maryland and associated Veterans Affairs system and now out of Massachusetts General Hospital and the Harvard University programs, over the past several years. In the following sections, we summarize the contributions of these leaders in the field in the context of lung xenotransplantation.

## NATURE OF THE PROBLEM

In broad terms, there are two separate issues that need to be addressed. First, there is a shortage of human donor lung allografts that is contributing to the high rates of morbidity and mortality among patients who are candidates for lung transplantation. Second, as it applies to addressing this organ shortage, clinically viable xenotransplantation of the lung lags significantly behind that for other organ systems in both experimental models and its clinical application because of the biological hurdles we have yet to overcome. The shortage of human donor allografts has dire consequences for patients on the waiting list because of low donor lung utilization of around 20%. Over the past 7 years, approximately 5%-7% of the lungs that were procured each year were not transplanted. Also, in 2020, approximately 10% of recipients waited 1 year or more for a lung transplant. Approximately, 17% of waitlisted candidates did not make it to transplant because they became too sick or died. The long waitlist times and the morbidity and mortality suffered while waiting for an organ to become available highlight the shortage of available organs and, more importantly, the consequences for the patients. Given that lung transplantation is the only viable therapeutic option for a number of end-stage lung pathologies, the waitlisted patients are left to await an organ that may never come. Meanwhile, they are suffering with their primary lung disease and the decreased quality of life associated with their illness.

Innovations in human lung allotransplantation that are intended to mitigate allograft shortages include expanding the donor pool with donation after cardiac death donors and assessing the injured human lung allograft using ex vivo lung perfusion strategies.[7] Although the technological advances that make ex vivo perfusion possible have the potential to increase the availability of donor lungs, barrier to their use include the short period of time for which the allografts can be placed safely on ex vivo lung perfusion, as well as their cost and logistical constraints at individual transplant centers.

In contrast to allotransplantation-based approaches to expanding the donor supply, xenotransplantation offers the exciting possibility of making the organ supply virtually unlimited and timely, as well as providing organs that are in an ideal clinical situation, physiologically appropriate, disease-free, and available locally (minimizing ischemia during transport). Although clinical lung xenotransplantation is likely years away, it would revolutionize human lung transplantation. Significant hurdles that need to be overcome are approachable with new tools in genetic engineering and other technologies. For example, the clustered regularly interspaced short palindromic repeats (CRISPR)/CRISPR-associated protein 9 (Cas9) technique, developed in 2014, has allowed rapid alteration of many genes in the donor animal. The commercialization of such advances has made it possible to more rapidly evaluate genetic modifications to lung xenografts. This has implications for experimental xenotransplantion to nonhuman primates, as well as for the use of ex vivo models.[7]

The lung is a complex organ, and several of its defining characteristics make it particularly vulnerable to injury following transplantation. One is its large vascular endothelial surface area, which sees the entire blood supply as it moves from the right to the left side of the heart. Others are its large epithelial surface area, its exposure to the external environment, the delicate nature of the pulmonary parenchyma, and its robust immune system (stimulates a strong host immune response).[7] Note that following pig-to-nonhuman primate xenotransplantation of both heart and kidney, function of the pig organs has been sustained for months,[8–12] yet in the case of lung xenografts, organ function has been limited to hours or days.

## RESEARCH

### *Immune Mechanisms*

In the genetically unaltered and medically untreated xenotransplantation models, injury comes, broadly, via two mechanisms: enhancement of blood coagulation and inflammation via activation of the complement system and the activities of preformed antibodies. These mechanisms lead to hyperacute rejection and associated graft failure within minutes. Early experimental genetic work in swine identified several carbohydrate antigens in the pig model that are not present in humans and significantly contribute to hyperacute rejection. These antigens, which are recognized by preformed antibodies in humans, include alpha 1,3-galactosyltransferase (Gal-T) gene. These antigens, which are recognized by preformed antibodies in humans, are carbohydrates added to proteins by the product of the *Gal-T* gene.[13–19]

Since these carbohydrate antigens were identified, research has focused on identifying mediators of lung xenograft injury, genetic modifications that address the coagulation cascade and immune barriers, and targets for drug therapies. The pig has become the preferred animal donor for organ xenotransplantation for several reasons. One is that pigs are easier to breed and house than nonhuman primates. In addition, the use of nonhuman primates as xenograft donors raises both ethical concerns and the risk of infection. Given that many of the advances in research on lung xenotransplantation are based largely on the pig xenograft donor, it is important to note some of the findings; they give a sense of complexity to xenograft tolerance and shed light on the likely future direction of the field.

One aspect of this complexity in xenograft tolerance relates to incompatibilities between receptors and their ligands. For example, having previously demonstrated that human macrophages are capable of phagocytosing pig cells and present a barrier to porcine-to-human xenotransplantation, Ide and colleagues,[20] using a real-time PCR assay, found that the signal regulatory protein (SIRP) alpha receptor in these cells is incompatible with the human form of its inhibitory ligand, CD47. Whereas in allografts, signaling between these proteins inhibits autologous phagocytosis of macrophages, and the protein sequence of the pig CD47 ligand suggested that it has limited compatibility with human macrophage SIRP alpha. Specifically, porcine CD47 did not induce SIRP alpha tyrosine phosphorylation in human macrophage-like cell lines. These authors demonstrated that interspecies incompatibility between SIRP alpha and CD47 significantly contributed to xenograft rejection by macrophages, specifically in porcine cells. These findings led them to propose that forced expression of human CD47 on porcine cells would create SIRP alpha-CD47 compatibility, preventing or at least repressing this particular mechanism of xenograft rejection.[20] More broadly, these findings highlight that interspecies incompatibilities between ligands and their receptors represent a series of molecular barriers to successful xenotransplantation, one that could affect multiple cellular functions including innate immune mechanisms and the coagulation cascade.

In 2017, French and colleagues published on the presentation of sialic acids and their central role in regulating inflammation and cell adhesion in the context of xenotransplantation.[21] This study identified several molecular targets for therapeutics; all of which were notable components of the sialic acid pathway.[21] The following year, the same group demonstrated, using an ex vivo pig lung perfusion experiment, that xenografting causes an increase in human interleukin (IL)-8 levels and associated activation of human neutrophils. The effect measured was increased adhesion neutrophils to pig aortic endothelial cells. This study implicated IL-8 as a mediator of lung inflammation and injury, supporting its potential as a therapeutic target in lung xenotransplantation.[22]

In the same year, Laird and colleagues studied 37 Gal 1,3-αGal antigen knockout (GalTKO) and human membrane cofactor protein (hCD46)-expressing (GalTKO.hCD46) pig lungs, comparing them to lungs of the same genetic background but modified to express the natural killer (NK) cell inhibitory ligand HLA-E (GalTKO.hCD46.HLA-E).[23] The xenografts were perfused ex vivo with human blood, and hemodynamics of the pulmonary artery and airway pressure were studied in real time. The authors also performed a cytotoxicity assay on porcine GalTKO.hCD46 aortic endothelial cells cultured with human NK cells, and they found that the expression of HLA-E on the former was associated with a decrease in NK-mediated cytotoxicity and an increase in median survival from 162 minutes to over 4 hours. They concluded that expression of HLA-E on GalTKO.hCD46 pig aortic endothelial cells is protective in the presence of human blood and that the activation of NK cells contributes to injury of these cells.[23] In this experiment, prefusion of the lung with human blood was terminated at 4 hours if the ex vivo lung did not fail. However, this once again emphasizes the limited graft survival of lung xenografts, measured in hours.

Much of the work on effects of preformed antibodies in humans on xenografts has been done by the Pierson group. This group evaluates antibody-mediated rejection by identifying and altering epitopes to which humans have preformed antibodies. In October 2022, they demonstrated that an ex vivo pig lung perfusion model with an additional N-Glycolylneuraminic acid knockout had significantly reduced antibody-mediated inflammation, as well as reduced activation of the coagulation cascade. These findings suggest that knocking out this gene would promote the success of lung xenografts in human recipients.[24]

### Coagulation Cascade Mechanisms

Activation of the coagulation pathway in the context of pig-human xenotransplantation has been attributed to incompatibilities between components of not only the inflammatory pathways but also the coagulation cascade. For example, the effect of the porcine tissue factor pathway inhibitor on human Factor Xa is thought to be weaker than that of its human counterpart. Similarly, the combination of pig thrombomodulin and human thrombin appears to more weakly activate protein C than the human-human pair does.[7,25,26] These coagulation-cascade incompatibilities represent another set of biological barriers to clinically viable lung xenotransplantation.

As recently suggested by the Burdorf and Pierson group, clinically viable lung xenotransplantation will likely require targeted drug therapies that minimize the effects of the intense inflammatory response to lung xenografts. The Burdorf and Pierson group, as well as Cantu and collegues,[27,28] had demonstrated long ago that in pigs, liposomal clodronate depletes lung-resident macrophages and attenuates hyperacute rejection. Since then, 1-benzylimidazole has been used to inhibit thromboxane synthase, and blockers of histamine receptors have been shown to attenuate the inflammatory response, reduce pulmonary vascular resistance, and reduce airway pressure.[27] More recent studies have focused on the upregulation and roles of integrins and selectins as cell adhesion molecules during inflammation.[7]

### Animal Models

The 2007 report by Cantu and colleagues[29] demonstrated the longest survival of a pig-to-nonhuman primate lung xenograft at the time. The most recent in vivo studies of pig-to-nonhuman primate lung xenotransplantation have used the baboon as the recipient. Even as more genetically engineered pig models have become available over the past few years, the baboon has continued to be the favored recipient for in vivo studies.

Recently, Burdorf and colleagues demonstrated extended survival of pig-to-baboon lung xenografts, with one recipient having survived 31 days.[12] This was accomplished using a series of genetic modifications and targeted therapies. Specifically, xenograft survival was prolonged when human endothelial protein C receptor and human thrombomodulin were expressed in the GalTKO.hCD46 pig and when the xenograft was treated with a combination of anti-inflammatory drugs that inhibit cytokines, blockers of selectins and integrins, and modulators of other mechanisms such as the depletion of donor lung macrophages.[12] Despite the limitations of this study in the context of human lung xenotransplantation, it demonstrates the significant advances that have been made in identifying and addressing the mechanisms that underlie tolerance to xenotransplantation. It is a promising report and demonstrates significant progress toward clinically viable human lung xenotransplantation.

### Alternative Xenogeneic Strategies

Another pig-human cross-species, or xenogeneic, lung model that was developed as a multi-institutional project over the past 3 years is worth mentioning, even though it does not fall strictly into the category of lung xenotransplantation. It uses pig xenogeneic cross-circulation to support and recover human donor lungs ex vivo, that is, preserving and even restoring lungs that would otherwise be unusable for human lung allografts. The concept expands on the principles of ex vivo lung perfusion, adding immune modulation, substrate metabolism, circulating repair factors, biochemical regulation, and metabolic clearance.[30] This approach has been shown to lead to significantly reduced inflammation as well as improved lung function and recovery times. For example, the typical limit for ischemia in lungs to be used in human allografts is approximately 6 hours. However, using procured human lungs already deemed unsuitable for transplantation that had sustained an average cold ischemic time of 20 hours, they demonstrated improved physiology. Immunosuppression and recombinant cobra venom were used to limit immune responses and compliment activation, respectively. After 24 hours of xenogeneic cross-circulation gas exchange, lung compliance, peak inspiratory pressure, and mean composite injury all significantly improved.[31,32]

As this model applies to the transplantation of human lung allografts, infectious and ethical concerns remain, as mentioned below. Practical barriers to applying these methods in standard practice are also considerable, and specialized organ recovery centers may be required. Nevertheless, the observed improvements in human lung allografts that had undergone prolonged cold ischemia suggests that this approach may be a viable platform for developing strategies to personalize lung allografts or xenografts before transplantation. Specifically, immunomodification, cell therapy, gene therapy, or cell-replacement therapy might benefit from the use of xenogeneic cross-circulation before transplantation to the human recipient.

## CASE REPORTS

To date, there are no reports of lung xenotransplantation into humans.

## CONCERNS

### Infectious Concerns

Although pig cells are resistant to some of the microorganisms of primary concern in human lung allografts (human immunodeficiency virus, human cytomegalovirus, hepatitis B, and hepatitis C), the possibility of animal-to-human transmission of some microorganisms remains an ongoing concern. For example, both porcine endogenous retroviruses (PERVs) and porcine circoviruses recently received attention related to their potential for pig-to-human transmission in the context of xenotransplantation.[3,33,34] The susceptibility of these viruses to inhibitors of retroviruses demonstrated that these inhibitors have potent activity against PERV replication.[35] Also, CRISPR-Cas9-mediated genome-wide inactivation of the 62 PERV copies in a particular porcine cell line resulted in a >1000-fold reduction in transmission of PERV to human cells.[36] Moreover, two separate reports demonstrated that PERV is not transmitted to nonhuman primates with corneal transplants or in a separate study of eight humans transplanted with porcine islet cells.[37,38] Porcine circovirus type 2 is known to cause severe disease in pigs but is not known to cause disease in immunocompetent humans, yet it has been recommended that the virus be eliminated from pigs before the use for xenotransplantation. The virus is thought to affect the monocyte and macrophage cell lines, and it is present in alveolar epithelial cells and vascular endothelium.[39] One recommended means of preventing transmission of pathogenic microorganisms to humans in the setting of xenotransplantation is the use of designated pathogen-free breeding colonies and regularly screening the animals. A list of pathogens not permitted in swine with a designated pathogen-free status has been proposed, and a number of assays to assess the colonies are available.[40]

### Ethical Concerns

Ethical concerns also relate to the use of xenografts for lung transplantation in humans. The following questions that have resurfaced and led to vigorous debate since the January 2022 pig-to-human cardiac xenotransplantation: how to conduct human trials; whether initial studies should be done on brain-dead recipients; when to begin clinical trials in living human recipients; who will be the first recipients; and how the first recipients will be selected. Additional ethical debates relate to how informed consent will be obtained, how the field will be regulated, and how data will be shared. Additional barriers include other regulatory issues and the fact that the costs of xenotransplantation will be considerable. Governing agencies and insurers will likely require clear definitions of the criteria for xenotransplantation, as well as expect outcomes comparable to those for human allografts. As the field evolves, it will also be necessary to resolve who will have oversight over allograft allocation and who will accredit xenotransplantation centers. The issue of when to begin clinical trials and the data reporting on them will likely be very important in the coming years. Caplan and colleagues have suggested that regulations require that all xenografts using genetically altered organs be performed after obtaining approval from institutional review boards and when protocols are standardized. Finally, the success of clinical lung xenotransplantation will require effective and timely sharing of findings.[41]

## DISCUSSION

The shortage of human lung allografts available for donation is not likely to be resolved by measures, already being used, to expand the human lung allograft pool. Addressing this donor organ shortage has focused intensive efforts on xenotransplantation. As is evidenced by the current state of research in solid organ xenotransplantation, the future of clinically viable human lung xenotransplantation is currently focused on the pig as a xenograft donor. There are several practical reasons for this, and as the pig has remained the favored model over the past few decades, significant progress has been made in identifying the biological barriers to transplanting the pig lung into a human recipient. Nevertheless, because the lung is particularly vulnerable to immunological insults, progress in xenotransplantation of this organ has lagged behind that of others. Notably, no human lung xenotransplantation has been reported, whereas in recent decades, significant progress has been made in pig-to-human xenotransplantation of both kidney and heart.

The innate vulnerabilities of the lung require that we identify the biological barriers to lung xenotransplantation, and current genetic engineering tools have provided the most recent means to both identify and overcome these barriers.

Recently developed animal models have led to significant and exciting progress in lung xenotransplantation in the laboratory but has done so with limited clinical application to human lung xenograft. In addition, issues related to cross-species infection, ethics, and regulatory issues remain to be addressed as xenotransplantation of other solid organs are becoming a clinical reality. In particular, a transparent approach to informed consent and data sharing will be critical to the success of the field.

## SUMMARY

Accomplishing clinically viable human lung xenotransplantation will require overcoming significant challenges. However, the shortage of lung allografts has pushed the field to consider alternatives to traditional lung allografts including high-risk donors, marginal allografts, and even xenotransplantation. Although xenotransplantation of the lung lags significantly behind that of other organs, research over the past several years has led to significant progress, and if successful, it has the potential to address organ shortage. Although valid concerns regarding cross-species transmission of pathogens raise ethical issues, new genetic engineering tools that are at our disposal have led to progress in identifying therapeutic targets and limit transmission of viruses. Finally, although lung xenotransplantation has not yet been reported, the development of pig-to-nonhuman primate models of lung xenotransplantation represents quantifiable progress in graft survival.

## CLINICS CARE POINTS

- The donor lung allograft shortage is not likely to be addressed, but currently efforts are made to expand the human lung allograft donor pool.
- Biological barriers to lung xenotransplantation are likely to be overcome, but this will require further research.
- The success of pig-to-human lung xenografts depends on studies being well planned and well executed.
- These studies must address all ethical considerations and be performed according to strict protocols.
- As human lung xenotransplantation moves toward clinical trials, data sharing will be critical to the success of the field.

## DISCLOSURE

The authors have nothing to disclose.

## REFERENCES

1. Valapour M, Lehr CJ, Skeans MA, et al, Organ Procurement and Transplantation Network (OPTN) and Scientific Registry of Transplant Recipients (SRTR). OPTN/SRTR 2020 Annual Data Report: Lung. Am J Transplant 2022;22(2):438–518.
2. Keeshan BC, Rossano JW, Beck N, et al. Lung transplant waitlist mortality: height as a predictor of poor outcomes. Pediatr Transplant 2015;19(3):294–300.
3. Ekser B, Li P, Cooper DKC. Xenotransplantation: past, present, and future. Curr Opin Organ Transplant 2017;22(6):513–21.
4. Hardy JD, Kurrus FD, Chavez CM, et al. Heart transplantation in man. Developmental studies and report of a case. JAMA 1964;188:1132–40.
5. Cooper DKC, Ekser B, Tector AJ. A brief history of clinical xenotransplantation. Int J Surg 2015;23(Pt B):205–10.
6. Chaban R, Cooper DKC, Pierson RN 3rd. Pig heart and lung xenotransplantation: present status. J Heart Lung Transplant 2022;41(8):1014–22.
7. Burdorf L, Azimzadeh AM, Pierson RN 3rd. Progress and challenges in lung xenotransplantation: an update. Curr Opin Organ Transplant 2018;23(6):621–7.
8. Mohiuddin MM, Singh AK, Corcoran PC, et al. One-year heterotopic cardiac xenograft survival in a pig to baboon model. Am J Transplant 2014;14(2):488–9.
9. Higginbotham L, Mathews D, Breeden CA, et al. Pre-transplant antibody screening and anti-CD154 costimulation blockade promote long-term xenograft survival in a pig-to-primate kidney transplant model. Xenotransplantation 2015;22(3):221–30.
10. Iwase H, Liu H, Wijkstrom M, et al. Pig kidney graft survival in a baboon for 136 days: longest life-supporting organ graft survival to date. Xenotransplantation 2015;22(4):302–9.
11. Langin M, Mayr T, Reichart B, et al. Consistent success in life-supporting porcine cardiac xenotransplantation. Nature 2018;564(7736):430–3.
12. Burdorf L, Laird CT, Harris DG, et al. Pig-to-baboon lung xenotransplantation: extended survival with targeted genetic modifications and pharmacologic treatments. Am J Transplant 2022;22(1):28–45.
13. Gonzalez-Stawinski GV, Daggett CW, Lau CL, et al. Non-anti-Gal alpha1-3Gal antibody mechanisms are sufficient to cause hyperacute lung dysfunction in pulmonary xenotransplantation. J Am Coll Surg 2002;194(6):765–73.
14. Phelps CJ, Koike C, Vaught TD, et al. Production of alpha 1,3-galactosyltransferase-deficient pigs. Science 2003;299(5605):411–4.

15. Chen G, Qian H, Starzl T, et al. Acute rejection is associated with antibodies to non-Gal antigens in baboons using Gal-knockout pig kidneys. Nat Med 2005;11(12):1295–8.
16. Nguyen BN, Azimzadeh AM, Zhang T, et al. Life-supporting function of genetically modified swine lungs in baboons. J Thorac Cardiovasc Surg 2007; 133(5):1354–63.
17. Byrne GW, Stalboerger PG, Davila E, et al. Proteomic identification of non-Gal antibody targets after pig-to-primate cardiac xenotransplantation. Xenotransplantation 2008;15(4):268–76.
18. Byrne GW, Stalboerger PG, Du Z, et al. Identification of new carbohydrate and membrane protein antigens in cardiac xenotransplantation. Transplantation 2011;91(3):287–92.
19. Nguyen BN, Azimzadeh AM, Schroeder C, et al. Absence of Gal epitope prolongs survival of swine lungs in an ex vivo model of hyperacute rejection. Xenotransplantation 2011;18(2):94–107.
20. Ide K, Wang H, Tahara H, et al. Role for CD47-SIRPalpha signaling in xenograft rejection by macrophages. Proc Natl Acad Sci U S A 2007;104(12): 5062–6.
21. French BM, Sendil S, Pierson RN 3rd, et al. The role of sialic acids in the immune recognition of xenografts. Xenotransplantation 2017;24(6):e12345.
22. French BM, Sendil S, Sepuru KM, et al. Interleukin-8 mediates neutrophil-endothelial interactions in pig-to-human xenogeneic models. Xenotransplantation 2018;25(2):e12385.
23. Laird CT, Burdorf L, French BM, et al. Transgenic expression of human leukocyte antigen-E attenuates GalKO.hCD46 porcine lung xenograft injury. Xenotransplantation 2017;24(2).
24. Chaban R, Habibabady Z, Hassanein W, et al. Knock-out of N-glycolylneuraminic acid attenuates antibody-mediated rejection in xenogenically perfused porcine lungs. Xenotransplantation 2022; 29(6):e12784.
25. Kopp CW, Siegel JB, Hancock WW, et al. Effect of porcine endothelial tissue factor pathway inhibitor on human coagulation factors. Transplantation 1997;63(5):749–58.
26. Roussel JC, Moran CJ, Salvaris EJ, et al. Pig thrombomodulin binds human thrombin but is a poor cofactor for activation of human protein C and TAFI. Am J Transplant 2008;8(6):1101–12.
27. Collins BJ, Blum MG, Parker RE, et al. Thromboxane mediates pulmonary hypertension and lung inflammation during hyperacute lung rejection. J Appl Physiol (1985) 2001;90(6):2257–68.
28. Cantu E, Gaca JG, Palestrant D, et al. Depletion of pulmonary intravascular macrophages prevents hyperacute pulmonary xenograft dysfunction. Transplantation 2006;81(8):1157–64.
29. Cantu E, Balsara KR, Li B, et al. Prolonged function of macrophage, von Willebrand factor-deficient porcine pulmonary xenografts. Am J Transplant 2007;7(1):66–75.
30. Hozain AE, O'Neill JD, Pinezich MR, et al. Xenogeneic cross-circulation for extracorporeal recovery of injured human lungs. Nat Med 2020;26(7): 1102–13.
31. Kelly Wu W, Guenthart BA, O'Neill JD, et al. Technique for xenogeneic cross-circulation to support human donor lungs ex vivo. J Heart Lung Transplant 2022;42(3):335–44.
32. O'Neill JD, Guenthart BA, Hozain AE, et al. Xenogeneic support for the recovery of human donor organs. J Thorac Cardiovasc Surg 2022;163(4): 1563–70.
33. Denner J, Mueller NJ. Preventing transfer of infectious agents. Int J Surg 2015;23(Pt B):306–11.
34. Denner J. Recent progress in xenotransplantation, with emphasis on virological safety. Ann Transplant 2016;21:717–27.
35. Argaw T, Colon-Moran W, Wilson C. Susceptibility of porcine endogenous retrovirus to anti-retroviral inhibitors. Xenotransplantation 2016;23(2):151–8.
36. Yang L, Guell M, Niu D, et al. Genome-wide inactivation of porcine endogenous retroviruses (PERVs). Science 2015;350(6264):1101–4.
37. Choi HJ, Kim J, Kim JY, et al. Long-term safety from transmission of porcine endogenous retrovirus after pig-to-non-human primate corneal transplantation. Xenotransplantation 2017;24(4).
38. Morozov VA, Wynyard S, Matsumoto S, et al. No PERV transmission during a clinical trial of pig islet cell transplantation. Virus Res 2017;227:34–40.
39. Denner J, Mankertz A. Porcine Circoviruses and Xenotransplantation. Viruses 2017;9(4):83. p. 1-13.
40. Fishman JA. Risks of infectious disease in Xenotransplantation. N Engl J Med 2022;387(24): 2258–67.
41. Caplan A, Parent B. Ethics and the emerging use of pig organs for xenotransplantation. J Heart Lung Transplant 2022;41(9):1204–6.

# Thermoablative Techniques to Treat Excessive Central Airway Collapse

Sidhu P. Gangadharan, MD, MHCM*, Fleming Mathew, MBBS

**KEYWORDS**

• Thermal ablation • Tracheobronchomalacia • Excessive central airway collapse
• Excessive dynamic airway collapse • Laser tracheobronchoplasty • Argon plasma coagulation

**KEY POINTS**

- Excessive central airway collapse refers to a reduction of over 70% cross-sectional area of the central airway lumen, which can result from various disease processes that affect the cartilage, the smooth muscles in the posterior wall, or both.
- The standard of care at our institution is to give the patient endobronchial stent-trial to establish candidacy for surgical correction. If the patient meets the criteria, tracheobronchoplasty is offered.
- Thermal ablation appears to be an experimental but potentially promising modality to be used in certain cases of ECAC.

## BACKGROUND

Excessive central airway collapse (ECAC) is characterized by an excessive narrowing of the trachea and mainstem bronchi during expiration. It encompasses two distinct disorders, namely, Tracheobronchomalacia (TBM) and Excessive Dynamic Airway Collapse (EDAC). TBM results from the weakening of the anterior cartilaginous rings, while EDAC is characterized by the excessive invagination of the posterior membrane of the trachea due to atrophy of trachealis smooth muscle fibers.[1] Both pathologic entities, when severe, may result in loss of airway lumen with expiration or other maneuvers which may cause positive intrapleural pressure (eg, coughing, laughing, speaking). On the basis of inheritance, Excessive central airway collapse can be broadly categorized into 2 types, *primary* (or *congenital*) and *secondary* (or *acquired*).

## PRIMARY OR CONGENITAL

a. *Presenting in childhood:* Etiology can vary from idiopathic to being associated with underlying primary syndromes such as Ehler-Danlos, bronchopulmonary dysplasia, DiGeorge and Hunter's syndrome.[2–4] In the pediatric population, ECAC exhibits nonspecific symptoms, such as a barking cough with expiratory rhonchi or inspiratory stridor, which depend on the location, extent, and severity of airway collapse. ECAC is often associated with other medical conditions, including esophageal atresia, tracheoesophageal fistula, and congenital heart disease. Diagnosis of TBM is usually achieved through direct visualization by flexible and rigid endoscopy and multidetector computed tomography (MDCT). Medical management focuses on optimizing ciliary clearance of secretions while awaiting airway structural stability. Surgical options depend on airway anatomy and pathology and include pexy procedures, tracheal resection and end-to-end anastomosis, and placement of external splints and internal stents.[5–7]
b. *Presenting in adulthood:* Mounier-Kuhn syndrome is a hereditary disorder that is inherited

Division of Thoracic Surgery and Interventional Pulmonology, Beth Israel Deaconess Medical Center, W/DC 201, 185 Pilgrim Road, Boston, MA 02215, USA
* Corresponding author.
*E-mail address:* sgangadh@bidmc.harvard.edu

Thorac Surg Clin 33 (2023) 299–308
https://doi.org/10.1016/j.thorsurg.2023.04.016

in an autosomal recessive pattern. It is characterized by the atrophy of the smooth muscles in the posterior wall of the trachea and bronchi, leading to tracheobronchial dilation. Symptoms typically appear during the third or fourth decade of life and vary widely in severity, from mild to severe respiratory failure and death. Diagnosis is typically made using CT scans, which can identify abnormally large air passages. Asymptomatic patients generally require no specific treatment, while symptomatic patients may benefit from supportive therapy such as respiratory physiotherapy and antibiotics during exacerbations. Although tracheal stenting can help in severe cases, surgery is seldom performed due to the diffuse nature of the disease. Lung transplantation has not been shown to improve the risk of morbidity and mortality.[8,9]

### *Secondary or Acquired*

a. *Secondary to injury or damage:* Chronic inflammation in COPD and asthma leads to the atrophy of the tracheobronchial wall, which is postulated to result in ECAC.[10] Additionally, tracheal cartilage injury caused by tuberculosis, progressive atrophy, and destruction of tracheal or bronchial cartilages due to recurrent polychondritis, as well as chronic inflammation and irritation from smoking or air pollution, may also contribute to the development of TBM.[11] Medical procedures such as prolonged tracheotomy and endotracheal intubation can result in pressure necrosis leading to injury of the central airways. Tracheal and bronchial malacia have also been observed in patients undergoing heart and lung transplantation. The cause of this complication is believed to be associated with certain suturing methods and lung preservation techniques.[12–16] In some cases, endobronchial electrosurgery used to treat lung cancer may result in cartilage damage, leading to tracheobronchomalacia.[17,18]
b. *Arising from chronic compression of central airways:* Pre-tracheal masses such as goiter, thymic or bronchogenic cyst, and various other mediastinal tumors may lead to tracheal compression. Other contributing factors that can lead to compression and, subsequently, ECAC include vascular anomalies such as vascular rings, malformations such as double aortic arch and right aortic arch with aberrant left subclavian vessel, post-pneumonectomy syndrome, dilated cardiomyopathy and severe scoliosis.[17,19]

## HISTOLOGY

There are limited postmortem data available on patients with ECAC. In our institution, we conducted a study of 14 tracheal specimens from patients diagnosed with tracheobronchomalacia (TBM) and tracheal stenosis (TS), which were then compared to normal tracheal specimens obtained from autopsy cases. Our findings revealed that both TBM and TS patients exhibited submucosal fibrotic changes. TBM patients also demonstrated alterations in the quality and density of elastin fibers in the posterior membrane. Additionally, we observed the upregulation of gene signatures in both proremodeling and proinflammatory pathways in the resected tracheal tissue of TBM patients, including FGFBP2, FGFR3, TGF$\beta$1, and TIMP1. While other proinflammatory markers such as TNF, IL1$\beta$, and IFN$\gamma$ did not reach statistical significance, they were still present. Histopathologic evaluation of TBM and TS samples showed connective tissue alterations and attenuation in the tracheal posterior wall when compared to specimens from autopsy control subjects.[20]

*Prevalence:* The absence of a standardized diagnostic criterion for tracheobronchomalacia (TBM) or excessive dynamic airway collapse (EDAC) in relation to the degree of central airway collapse has resulted in variations in cut-off values for the percentage loss of cross-sectional area, thus impeding accurate determination of the prevalence of expiratory central airway collapse (ECAC). Nonetheless, existing literature suggests a prevalence range of 4% to 23% among patients who undergo bronchoscopy for various indications.[17] In However, primary ECAC is a frequent occurrence in the pediatric demographic, and its prevalence among children is approximately 1 in 2100.[5]

## DIAGNOSIS

*Signs and Symptoms:* Patients often present with nonspecific symptoms such as breathlessness, inability to clear airway secretions, cough, and gastroesophageal reflux. These clinical features are similar to those observed in patients with COPD or asthma. However, patients with ECAC may have a characteristic seal-like barking cough which may arise due to a compliant central airway vibrating during a forced exhalation or cough. A physical examination may exhibit wheezing, rhonchi, reduced breath sounds, or inadequate air movement.[17]

*Diagnosis criteria*: Dynamic flexible bronchoscopy (DFB) is currently considered the most reliable method for diagnosing TBM. It allows the real-time examination of the airways and provides accurate information on dynamic airway properties. Dynamic expiratory CT is also highly sensitive in detecting airway collapse. This noninvasive test has been found to be concordant with DFB in detecting airway malacia. Dynamic expiratory CT provides a detailed image of the airways during expiration, allowing for the identification of malacic segments in the airways. According to Ruiz and colleagues,[21] the interrater reliability of CT and DFB in diagnosing airway collapse is not optimal. The authors recommend that both tests be used, as omitting one test or the other could result in misdiagnosis of TBM. Unlike most literature on ECAC, which defines the presence of disease using a cut-off of 50% decrease in cross-sectional area of the airway lumen, our findings consistently reveal that a significant proportion of healthy volunteers experience airway collapse exceeding 50% of cross sectional area during cough maneuvers or expiration.[22] Hence, in our institution, we define ECAC to be a collapse of central airways exceeding 70%, which correlates well with symptoms. We classify 70% as mild, 80% to 89% as moderate, and greater than 90% as severe collapse.

Pulmonary function tests (PFT) are primarily used to evaluate pulmonary comorbidity and predict the likelihood of a difficult recovery after tracheobronchoplasty since PFT values do not correlate well with the severity of TBM.[23–25] Before surgical evaluation, patients are commonly evaluated for vocal cord dysfunction and gastroesophageal reflux disease (GERD), which require adequate treatment if present. Physiologic assessment, including a 6-min walk test, is also conducted, and standardized questionnaires are administered to assess functional status using the Karnofsky Performance Scale, modified Medical Research Council (mMRC) dyspnea scale, and quality of life using St. George Respiratory Questionnaire (SGRQ) and Cough Specific Quality of Life Questionnaire (CQLQ).[26]

*Standard of care:* When severe, diffuse tracheobronchomalacia (TBM) is diagnosed and found to cause significant symptoms and reduced quality of life, treatment is considered. At our institution, self-expanding metal stents or a Y-shaped silicone tracheobronchial stent aare placed to determine if the patient is a candidate for surgical intervention. After a 2-week trial period, patients are evaluated in the clinic to assess the degree of improvement in symptomatology resulting from the stabilization of the central airways. Those who show marked improvement are considered for definitive surgical intervention. This approach provides valuable prognostic information on the patient's response to surgery.[22]

Tracheobronchoplasty involves suturing a polypropylene mesh to the posterior membrane of the tracheobronchial tree.[27] The careful sizing of the prosthesis and the precise placement of sutures to the airway yields excellent results with regard to short and long-term anatomic, symptomatic, and functional outcomes.[25,28,29]

## THERMOABLATIVE TECHNIQUES

### *Background*

Thermal ablation using lasers is an emerging treatment option for many abdominal and thoracic neoplasms that are resistant to conventional therapies. During a thermal ablation procedure, a thin applicator is guided into the target site using bronchoscopic guidance. The tissue is then subjected to energy until temperatures reach cytotoxic levels.[30,31] The effects of heat on biological tissue are influenced not only by the temperature achieved but also by the duration and rate of heating. Therefore, understanding the multifaceted impact of heating on tissue is crucial in comprehending the biological response to thermal treatments.

Lasers interact with biological tissue through a combination of different tissue and laser parameters. Tissue parameters include optical and thermal properties such as reflection, absorption, scattering, and heat conduction while laser parameters include wavelength, exposure time, energy, spot size, and power density. Among the various interactions between lasers and tissue, 2 important reactions are "photobiomodulation" and "photothermal" reactions.

Photobiomodulation refers to chemical reactions in which a photon emitted by a light source modulates cellular behavior. Cytochrome c oxidase, a commonly studied photosensitizer within the cell, absorbs photons and increases the levels of reactive oxygen species (ROS), which triggers transcription factors for cellular repair. The enzyme also mediates the release of nitric oxide (NO), a vasodilator that increases cellular circulation. Photothermal reactions occur when tissues are exposed to temperatures that can cause either coagulation, vaporization, carbonization, or melting. The lowest temperatures by which biological tissue is thermally affected range from approximately 42 to 50°C. Beyond 50°C, an impedance of biochemical reactions within the cell is observed due to enzyme inactivation. At 60°C, denaturation of proteins and collagen leads to tissue coagulation and cell necrosis. Beyond 80°C, membrane permeability increases and results in the destruction of the cell. At 100°C, water molecules start to vaporize, which is beneficial since the vapor generated carries away excess heat and helps prevent further temperature increase in adjacent tissue. The biological impact of lasers is determined by the interaction between the level of cellular stimulation and the degree of tissue denaturation. When appropriately calibrated, lasers can activate cytochrome c oxidase, which, in turn, promotes cellular repair by activating transcription factors. However, excessive laser fluence can damage the cell and undo this function. Studies have shown that photothermal reactions are influenced not only by the temperature attained but also by the duration of tissue exposure to laser treatment.[32]

In the context of ECAC, surgical airway stabilization via tracheobronchoplasty (TBP) remains the standard of care for patients with severe symptomatic ECAC. However, TBP does carry risks of long-term complications such as chronic pain, disease recurrence requiring redo-TBP, dysphagia, and mesh erosion.[26] Hence, in this section, we want to provide an overview of the current research status on the use of bronchoscopic thermal ablation as a minimally invasive technique in the treatment of ECAC. We will focus on the efficacy and future directions of this experimental approach.

To start, we will provide a brief overview of the thermoablative techniques utilized by the authors in both animal models and human subjects to investigate their impact on ECAC, as referenced in our article.

1. Electrocautery: Electrocautery (EC) is a contact-based ablation technique that employs electric current flow to generate heat for tissue coagulation. The technique utilizes various types of unipolar electrodes, such as blunt probes, knives, forceps, and wire snare loops. However, the effectiveness of electrocautery largely depends on ensuring the essential contact of the electrode with the mucosa, which requires suctioning of secretion, blood, or debris at the site of treatment. The tissue effect of electrocautery is influenced by the wattage setting, the surface area of contact, with a smaller probe resulting in increased current density, and the duration of energy application. Monopolar electric current modalities can pose a limitation due to their potential interaction with pacemakers. Therefore, pacemakers must be inactivated prior to the commencement of the procedure.[33]
2. Argon plasma coagulation: Argon-plasma coagulation (APC) refers to a type of monopolar electrical coagulation that is noncontact in nature. It operates by utilizing argon gas as the conductive medium. Because APC is a noncontact method and has a lower energy density, it creates a superficial but more uniform thermal effect. APC adjusts the application of electrical energy based on the tissue's electrical conductivity. As the tissue's electrical conductivity decreases, the APC system searches for adjacent tissue that offers less electrical resistance. This results in a uniform depth of penetration, which is approximately 3 mm compared to EC with a penetration of ~ 4 to 8 mm. The APC technique thus provides uniform coagulation of the tissue and minimizes the risk of airway perforation.[34] Similar to EC, which is a monopolar technique, it is crucial to exercise caution in patients with pacemakers or automatic implantable cardioverter/defibrillators (AICDs), due to potential dysrhythmias or device malfunction. The device should be turned off whenever possible and clinically indicated.[35,36]
3. Radio-frequency ablation: Radiofrequency ablation (RFA) has become a popular alternative to surgical resection in the treatment of malignant tumors due to its minimally invasive nature and cost-effectiveness. RFA utilizes radiofrequency, an electromagnetic wave frequency, to destroy biological tissues by employing an unmodulated sinusoidal wave alternating current.[37] Monopolar RFA devices have a single active electrode that dissipates current through a grounding pad, while bipolar RFA devices have 2 active electrodes in close proximity, resulting in the destruction of intervening tissues without requiring a grounding pad.[38] Unlike electrocautery (EC), which employs an electrically heated tip to coagulate tissue and control bleeding, no RF current flows through the patient. Although case reports have suggested that RFA is safe in the presence of a pacemaker, caution should be exercised.[39,40] Compared to APC, RFA induces local thermal injury to tissues near the ablation site. While there have been reports of a sudden increase in patient temperature by 0.5°C to 2.3°C during RFA procedures, no other adverse effects have been observed as a result of this increase in body temperature.[41]
4. Laser techniques: In the following section, we explore several studies that have utilized various laser techniques including potassium-titanyl-phosphate (KTP), Holmium laser, and yttrium aluminum perovskite (YAP) laser to treat ECAC. The KTP laser emits green light, which has a strong affinity for both melanin and oxyhemoglobin. It has proven its efficacy in treating a diverse range of conditions, such as

vascular lesions, acne, verruca, and scars, among other dermatologic pathologies.[42] Recently, the Holmium laser has been utilized for transurethral resection of the prostate.[43] Moreover, the yttrium aluminum perovskite (YAP) laser has been safely used to reduce tumor size, alleviate tracheal stenosis, and manage excessive granulation tissue.[44]

## ANIMAL STUDIES

We sought to test the immediate effects of four different thermoablative methods (APC, RFA, EC, and KTP) on the airway wall using an ex vivo sheep model.[45] The study aimed to evaluate the feasibility of an ex vivo sheep model as a suitable alternative to study large airway disease. The sheep model was chosen because it shares a similar histologic distribution to humans. We found that APC at higher power settings demonstrated a consistent and homogenous thermal injury effect across all tissue layers, potentially allowing for future tissue regeneration and fibrosis (**Fig. 1**). The remaining treatment modalities produced a pattern of heterogenous thermal injury with areas of complete erosion and limited viable tissue for potential regeneration. Our study concluded that these methods should be further evaluated for their ability to induce airway fibrosis. It is also important to note that we used an ex vivo model that provides no tissue regenerative capacity. Hence, the medium and long-term effects of the different modalities, as well as their safety and reproducibility, could not be established. To address the limitations of the previous study we aimed to assess the postoperative changes and tissue regeneration in a live animal model.[46] Our objective this time was to evaluate the impact of argon plasma coagulation (APC) on tracheobronchial tissue in a living sheep model. Two male Dorset sheep underwent the procedure after a 7-day acclimation period, followed by a 30-day follow-up period during which a chest CT was obtained, and the sheep were monitored for clinical signs of pain, hemoptysis, infection, and respiratory difficulty. After the follow-up period, both sheep were intubated, and a flexible bronchoscopic evaluation was performed to visually assess the healing process of the trachea. The histologic findings were compared to those of 2 additional sheep cadavers. During the 30-day follow-up, the postprocedural chest CT scans showed no signs of complications, and there were no significant clinical events. At the 30-day follow-up bronchoscopy, the airways showed no stenotic segments, perforations, or evidence of infection. The tracheobronchial tissue displayed a complete reconstitution of the epithelium along the treated area, and the macroscopic appearance of the tissue was healthy, regardless of the power settings used. Microscopically, only minor surface epithelial changes were observed, ranging from squamous metaplasia to an attenuation of the normal ciliated bronchial epithelium. The submucosal smooth muscle layer remained intact with all applied treatment levels. However, there was a significant increase in the qualitative density and amount of fibroblastic collagen deposition in the targeted posterior membrane sites (**Fig. 2**). This study's limitations included a small sample size, the choice of healthy sheep without an airway collapse, and untreated controls. Nevertheless, this study was a milestone in providing histologic evidence after using APC to demonstrate its effect on collagen synthesis and tissue regeneration.

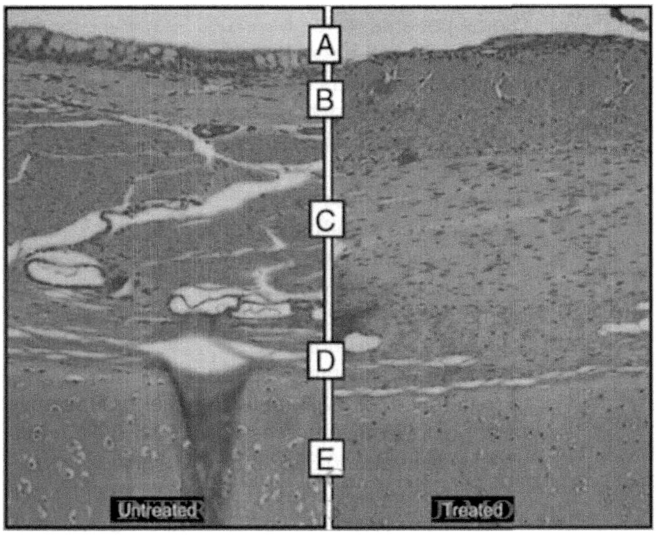


**Fig. 1.** In the examined layers of the trachea that is, epithelium (A), submucosa (B), smooth muscle (C), fibrous connective tissue (D), and cartilage (E), the treated tissue demonstrated changes consistent with acute thermal injury defined by the presence of surface (1) epithelium ablation, (2) elastic and collagen fiber condensation, (3) smooth muscle cells cytoplasm condensation with hypereosinophilic change, and (4) chondrocyte nuclei pyknosis. (*From* de Lima A, Vidal B, Kheir F, et al. Thermoablative Techniques for Excessive Central Airway Collapse: An Ex Vivo Pilot Study on Sheep Tracheal Tissue. J Bronchology Interv Pulmonol. 2020;27(3):195-199.)

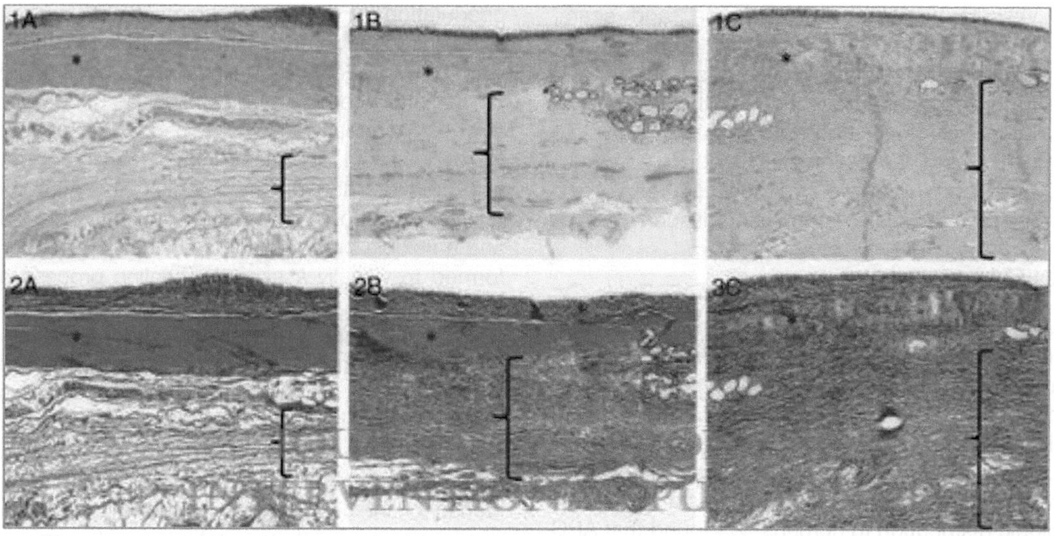


**Fig. 2.** Histopathology of treated segments of tracheal posterior membrane. (1) Hematoxylin and eosin stains (× 40 original magnification), (2) Trichrome stains (40 × original magnification). A, Effect 3. B, Effect 5. C, Effect 7. The density and overall thickness of the collagen fiber layer (blue staining on the trichrome stains) as highlighted by the brackets demonstrates a progressive increase in the posterior membrane that correlates with the escalating treatment effect intensity. This submucosal fibrosis is mainly observed beneath the smooth muscle layer (*asterisk*). (*From* Kheir F, Ospina-Delgado D, Beattie J, et al. Argon Plasma Coagulation (APC) for the Treatment of Excessive Dynamic Airway Collapse (EDAC): An Animal Pilot Study. J Bronchology Interv Pulmonol. 2021;28(3):221-227.)

## STUDIES IN HUMAN SUBJECTS

Castellanos and colleagues[47] conducted a retrospective analysis on 10 patients who underwent laser tracheobronchoplasty using holmium laser to treat excessive dynamic airway collapse (EDAC). The enrolled patients completed a Dyspnea Index (DI) questionnaire, which measured symptom severity on a scale from 0 to 40, where 0 indicated no symptoms and 40 indicated the presence of severe symptoms. The questionnaire was also administered 12 weeks after the operation. The mean score for the preoperative questionnaire was 35.7, with a range of 32 to 40, indicating that the patients experienced severe dyspnea. The procedure was performed while the patients were under general anesthesia, using a quartz fiber to deliver the laser via the operating channel of the bronchoscope. The laser was used to create deep furrows in the mucosal layer of the posterior wall of the tracheobronchial tree in a longitudinal, transverse, and serpentine manner from the distal to the proximal end while preserving intact mucosal areas in between the treated areas. The entire trachea, main stem, lobar, and segmental bronchi were treated, taking approximately 45 minutes for the procedure to complete. Two to 3 procedures were necessary to sufficiently stiffen the posterior tracheobronchial wall, with a 12-week interval between each stage required for sufficient tissue regeneration process. Copious saline irrigation was used to cleanse any blood and soft tissue debris from the airway, and no suction cautery was required for hemostasis during the procedure.

Following the procedure, patients were observed in a monitored setting for at least 48 hours to ensure proper airway function. They received respiratory care in the form of 3% sodium chloride to help clear secretions and IV antibiotics. Some patients were given 20% N-acetyl L-cystine along with half-strength albuterol sulfate to clear reactive secretions and sloughing tissue/eschar. Upon discharge, patients were prescribed oral antibiotics for a week and a nebulizer as and when needed. Patients were followed for more than 6 months after the procedure, during which time they showed significant improvement in their respiratory symptoms.

The postoperative mean Dyspnea Index score came out to be 12.5 with a range between 9 and 19. The results indicated a significant improvement in the patients' respiratory symptoms, with a difference of 23.3 between the preoperative and postoperative scores ($P < .001$, 95% confidence intervals: 20.38–26.02). No significant complications occurred in this series of patients, and on interval bronchoscopies after surgery, most had small tufts of granulation tissue that were easily suctioned away by the bronchoscope. No cases of cicatricial scarring in the trachea or mainstem were encountered. However, this study has some limitations. This includes a small sample size and a shorter follow-up period, which does not account for late complications or recurrences. Additionally, the authors defined EDAC as a loss of greater than 50% cross-sectional area of the central airways. The authors did not comment on the degree of collapse within the 10 patients who underwent laser tracheobronchoplasty. We define EDAC as a collapse of central airways resulting in the loss of greater than 70% of cross-sectional area at our center, since a significant number of healthy individuals have central airway collapse of greater than 50% without any accompanying signs or symptoms. So based on the results from this study, it is unclear whether patients with a higher degree of collapse would benefit from laser tracheobronchoplasty.

Dutau and colleagues[48] reported a case of successful management of Mounier-Kuhn syndrome using yttrium aluminum perovskite (YAP) laser. The patient, a 68-year-old woman, presented with complaints of chronic cough, occasional acute dyspnea, recurrent bouts of febrile illness and purulent sputum production, and audible wheezing. Imaging and bronchoscopic examination showed nearly complete collapse of the posterior tracheal membrane and the left mainstem bronchus during expiration. Rigid bronchoscopy with YAP laser treatment was performed to devascularize and retract the tissues in the posterior membrane. The patient experienced significant clinical improvement, which was supported by the postintervention pulmonary function tests and bronchoscopic examination results. A second treatment was performed 14 months later due to a slight recurrence of posterior membrane collapse, which remained asymptomatic. The patient received a total of 4 YAP laser procedures, but the frequency and reasons for these repeat procedures were not specified in the article. The patient was followed-up for 8 years and remained asymptomatic throughout this period. While the diagnosis of Mounier-Kuhn syndrome in this patient whose transverse tracheal diameter was only 26 mm may be questioned, the overall result anatomically and symptomatically appears to be very positive.

At our center, we recommend a stent-trial to determine if anatomic correction of the airways can alleviate symptoms before performing tracheobronchoplasty. However, complications may arise from endobronchial stents including stent fracture, migration, and airway obstruction due to inflammation and granulation tissue formation. Ching and colleagues[49] reported a case of a 43-year-old male with tracheomalacia resulting from inhalational injury. This patient received an uncovered nitinol endotracheal stent for malacic airways. The patient subsequently developed progressive tracheal stenosis caused by granulation tissue formation in and around the stent for which he received serial thermoablative procedures with APC. The stent however also fractured, causing metallic fragments to displace into the trachea. To address this issue, the team utilized APC to evaporate exposed metal while avoiding harm to surrounding structures. The patient responded well to these procedures, experiencing immediate relief of obstructive symptoms without any significant complication. Colt and colleagues[50] also describe a similar effect in their in vitro study on the use of APC around endobronchial stents. They described that short bursts of APC produced adequate tissue devitalization without igniting or rupturing the stent.

Plojoux and colleagues[51] conducted a single-center retrospective study on 60 patients with Dynamic A-Shape tracheal stenosis (DATS). DATS is defined as an anterior fracture of tracheal cartilage, which is often accompanied by posterior malacia. Among the 60 patients, 33 had posterior tracheomalacia. The authors carefully selected 5 patients with moderate stenosis and predominantly posterior localized malacia to utilize YAP (yttrium aluminum perovskite) for photocoagulation. The study reported a 100% success rate in treating the posterior localized malacia with YAP laser. However, the authors did not disclose how many times the laser procedure was repeated in the 5 patients, nor did they elaborate on the patient criteria they used to determine the suitability of YAP laser therapy versus endobronchial stent placement or surgery in the patients who received it. Furthermore, the study did not state the duration of patient follow-up after receiving the laser therapy, which is a crucial factor in evaluating the long-term effectiveness of the treatment.

## SUMMARY

Thermoablative bronchoscopic approaches have emerged as a potentially viable alternative to traditional tracheobronchoplasty for the treatment of excessive central airway collapse. Although limited to animal models and a few independent case reports and retrospective observational studies, the initial results of this experimental technique are promising. However, further research is necessary to evaluate the efficacy and safety of this approach in humans. As such, thermoablative techniques for EDAC should be considered experimental at this stage, and their use should be guided by careful consideration of the available evidence and individual patient circumstances.

## CLINICS CARE POINTS

- Excessive central airway collapse (ECAC) is characterized by excessive narrowing of trachea and mainstem bronchi during expiration. There are 2 subtypes of ECAC: Tracheobronchomalacia (TBM) and Excessive Dynamic Airway Collapse (EDAC). TBM occurs when the anterior cartilaginous rings weaken, while EDAC is characterized by excessive invagination of the posterior tracheal membrane due to the atrophy of trachealis smooth muscle fibers.
- The initial standard of care for central airway collapse involves addressing any underlying conditions such as asthma, COPD, and gastro-esophageal reflux. If medical treatment fails to improve severe symptoms, patients may be offered a stent-trial to determine if surgical correction of the obstruction is a viable option. If the stent-trial effectively resolves the patient's symptoms and the patient is deemed eligible for surgery, tracheobronchoplasty may be suggested as a definitive treatment approach.
- Based on preclinical studies, argon plasma coagulation (APC) appears to be one of the safest options for thermoablation. Studies indicate that APC can be safely used with indwelling endobronchial stents and provides even coagulation of tissue, reducing the risk of airway perforation.
- Currently reports of thermoablative approaches to treating ECAC in humans are limited to bronchoscopic laser treatments. The presumed mechanism of action is the formation of retractile scar in response to the controlled membranous wall injury created by the laser. Thermoablative bronchoscopic treatments may be a promising alternative to traditional tracheobronchoplasty for treating excessive central airway collapse. Although initial results in animal models and a few case reports and retrospective studies are encouraging, further research is needed to assess safety and effectiveness in humans. Thermoablative techniques are still experimental, and their use should be based on available evidence and individual patient needs.

## DISCLOSURE

The authors have nothing to disclose.

## REFERENCES

1. Janowiak P, Rogoza K, Siemińska A, et al. Expiratory central airway collapse – an overlooked entity?: Two case reports. Medicine 2020;99(42):E22449.
2. Wallis C, Alexopoulou E, Antón-Pacheco JL, et al. ERS statement on tracheomalacia and bronchomalacia in children. Eur Respir J 2019;54(3). https://doi.org/10.1183/13993003.00382-2019.
3. Huang RY, Shapiro NL. Structural airway anomalies in patients with DiGeorge syndrome: A current review. Am J Otolaryngol 2000;21(5):326–30.
4. Morehead JM, Parsons DS. Tracheobronchomalacia in Hunter's syndrome. Int J Pediatr Otorhinolaryngol 1993;26(3):255–61.
5. Boogaard R, Huijsmans SH, Pijnenburg MWH, et al. Tracheomalacia and bronchomalacia in children: incidence and patient characteristics. Chest 2005; 128(5):3391–7.
6. Jo Svetanoff W, Jennings RW. Mini review open access updates on surgical repair of tracheobronchomalacia. J Lung Health Dis 2018;2(1):17–23.
7. Kamran A, Jennings RW. Tracheomalacia and Tracheobronchomalacia in Pediatrics: An Overview of Evaluation, Medical Management, and Surgical Treatment. Front Pediatr 2019;7:512.
8. Celik B, Bilgin S, Yuksel C. Mounier-Kuhn Syndrome: A Rare Cause of Bronchial Dilation. Tex Heart Inst J 2011;38(2):194. Available at: http://pmc/articles/PMC3066798. Accessed February 25, 2023.
9. Menon B, Aggarwal B, Iqbal A. Mounier-Kuhn syndrome: report of 8 cases of tracheobronchomegaly with associated complications. South Med J 2008; 101(1):83–7.
10. Chetambath R. Tracheobronchomalacia in obstructive airway diseases. Lung India 2016;33(4):451.
11. Iwamoto Y, Miyazawa T, Kurimoto N, et al. Interventional Bronchoscopy in the Management of Airway Stenosis Due to Tracheobronchial Tuberculosis. Chest 2004;126(4):1344–52.
12. Airway Adversaries: Chronic Rejection and Tracheomalacia Following Lung Transplantation 2:30 pm — 3:50 pm. Chest 1995;108(3):122S–3S.
13. Crespo MM. Airway complications in lung transplantation. J Thorac Dis 2021;13(11):6717–24.
14. Salerno TA, Ontario C. The importance of acquired diffuse bronchomalacia in heart-lung transplant recipients with obliterative bronchiolitis. J Thorac Cardiovasc Surg 1991;101:643–8.
15. Novick RJ, Ahmad D, Menkis AH, et al. The importance of acquired diffuse bronchomalacia in heart-lung transplant recipients with obliterative bronchiolitis. J Thorac Cardiovasc Surg 1991;101(4):643–8.

16. Date H, Trulock EP, Arcidi JM, et al. Improved airway healing after lung transplantation: An analysis of 348 bronchial anastomoses. J Thorac Cardiovasc Surg 1995;110(5):1424–33.
17. Murgu SD, Colt HG. Tracheobronchomalacia and excessive dynamic airway collapse. Respirology 2006;11(4):388–406.
18. van Boxem TJM, Westerga J, Venmans BJW, et al. Tissue Effects of Bronchoscopic Electrocautery. Chest 2000;117(3):887–91.
19. Biswas A, Jantz MA, Sriram PS, et al. Tracheobronchomalacia. Dis Mon 2017;63(10):287–302.
20. Singh R, Vidal B, Ascanio J, et al. Pilot Gene Expression and Histopathologic Analysis of Tracheal Resections in Tracheobronchomalacia. Ann Thorac Surg 2022;114(5):1925–32.
21. Ruiz J, Somocurcio DE, Majid A, et al. Cardiothoracic Surgery SESSION TITLE: Cardiothoracic Surgery Posters SESSION TYPE: Original Investigation Posters BRONCHOSCOPY AND CT ARE NOT ALWAYS CONCORDANT WHEN USED TO EVALUATE TRACHEOBRONCHOMALACIA. Cardiothorac Surg 2020. https://doi.org/10.1016/j.chest.2020.08.097.
22. Gangadharan SP. Tracheobronchomalacia in Adults. Semin Thorac Cardiovasc Surg 2010;22(2):165–73.
23. Alape DE, Gangadharan S, Folch E, Folch A, Ochoa S, Majid A. Tracheobronchoplasty for Severe Tracheobronchomalacia: Short and Long-Term Outcomes. In: B39. INTERVENTIONAL PULMONARY MEDICINE: RECENT ADVANCES. American Thoracic Society International Conference Abstracts. American Thoracic Society; 2016:A3386-A3386. May 16, 2016. San Francisco, CA. doi:doi:10.1164/ajrccm-conference.2016.193.1_MeetingAbstracts. A3386.
24. Buitrago DH, Majid A, Alape DE, et al. Single-Center Experience of Tracheobronchoplasty for Tracheobronchomalacia: Perioperative Outcomes. Ann Thorac Surg 2018;106(3):909–15.
25. Majid A, Guerrero J, Gangadharan S, et al. Tracheobronchoplasty for severe tracheobronchomalacia: A prospective outcome analysis. Chest 2008; 134(4):801–7.
26. Buitrago DH, Wilson JL, Parikh M, et al. Current concepts in severe adult tracheobronchomalacia: evaluation and treatment. J Thorac Dis 2017;9(1):E57–66.
27. Gangadharan SP, Bakhos CT, Majid A, et al. Technical aspects and outcomes of tracheobronchoplasty for severe tracheobronchomalacia. Ann Thorac Surg 2011;91(5):1574–81.
28. Buitrago DH, Majid A, Wilson JL, et al. Tracheobronchoplasty yields long-term anatomy, function, and quality of life improvement for patients with severe excessive central airway collapse. J Thorac Cardiovasc Surg 2023;165(2):518–25.
29. Bezuidenhout AF, Boiselle PM, Heidinger BH, et al. Longitudinal follow-up of patients with tracheobronchomalacia after undergoing tracheobronchoplasty: Computed tomography findings and clinical correlation. J Thorac Imaging 2019;34(4):278–83.
30. Abtin FG, Eradat J, Gutierrez AJ, et al. Radiofrequency Ablation of Lung Tumors: Imaging Features of the Postablation Zone. Radiographics 2012; 32(4):947–69.
31. Shepherd RW, Radchenko C. Bronchoscopic ablatio techniques in the management of lung cancer. Ann Transl Med 2019;7(15):362.
32. Niemz Fundamentals MH. Laser-Tissue Interactions. Available at: https://link.springer.com/book/10.1007/978-3-540-72192-5#bibliographic-information.
33. Rosell A, Stratakos G. Therapeutic bronchoscopy for central airway diseases. Eur Respir Rev 2020; 29(158):1–10.
34. Morice RC, Ece T, Ece F, et al. Endobronchial argon plasma coagulation for treatment of hemoptysis and neoplastic airway obstruction. Chest 2001;119(3):781–7.
35. Bolliger C, Mathur Members P, Beamis J, et al. ERS/ATS statement on interventional pulmonology. Eur Respir J 2002;19(2):356–73.
36. Oberg C, Folch E, Santacruz JF. Management of malignant airway obstruction. AME Med J 2018; 3(0):115.
37. Ni Y, Mulier S, Miao Y, et al. A review of the general aspects of radiofrequency ablation. Abdom Imaging 2005;30(4):381–400.
38. McGahan JP, Gu WZ, Brock JM, et al. Hepatic ablation using bipolar radiofrequency electrocautery. Acad Radiol 1996;3(5):418–22.
39. Tong NY, Ru HJ, Ling HY, et al. Extracardiac Radiofrequency Ablation Interferes with Pacemaker Function but Does Not Damage the Device. Anesthesiology 2004;100(4):1041.
40. Hayes DL, Charboneau JW, Lewis BD, et al. Radiofrequency Treatment of Hepatic Neoplasms in Patients With Permanent Pacemakers. Mayo Clin Proc 2001;76(9):950–2.
41. Goodman EJ, Johnson PA. Radiofrequency ablation of hepatic tumors can cause elevation of the patient's temperature. Anesth Analg 2003;97(4):1203–4.
42. Green JB, Serowka K, Saedi N, et al. Potassium-Titanyl-Phosphate (KTP) Laser. 2014;1:66–76. doi: 10.1159/000355049.
43. Gilling PJ, Cass CB, Cresswell MD, et al. The use of the holmium laser in the treatment of benign prostatic hyperplasia. J Endourol 1996;10(5):459–61.
44. Lee HJ, Malhotra R, Grossman C, et al. Initial report of neodymium: Yttrium- aluminum-perovskite (Nd:YAP) laser use during bronchoscopy. J Bronchology Interv Pulmonol 2011;18(3):229–32.
45. de Lima A, Vidal B, Kheir F, et al. Thermoablative Techniques for Excessive Central Airway Collapse: An Ex Vivo Pilot Study on Sheep Tracheal Tissue. J Bronchology Interv Pulmonol 2020;27(3):195–9.
46. Kheir F, Ospina-Delgado D, Beattie J, et al. Argon Plasma Coagulation (APC) for the Treatment of

Excessive Dynamic Airway Collapse (EDAC): An Animal Pilot Study. J Bronchology Interv Pulmonol 2021;28(3):221–7.

47. Castellanos P, Mk M, Atallah I. Laser tracheobronchoplasty: a novel technique for the treatment of symptomatic tracheobronchomalacia. Eur Arch Oto-Rhino-Laryngol 2017;274(3):1601–7.

48. Dutau H, Maldonado F, Breen DP, et al. Endoscopic successful management of tracheobronchomalacia with laser: apropos of a Mounier-Kuhn syndrome. Eur J Cardio Thorac Surg 2011;39(6):e186–8.

49. Ching YH, Geck RD, Andrews AD, et al. Argon plasma coagulation in the management of uncovered tracheal stent fracture. Respir Med Case Rep 2014. https://doi.org/10.1016/j.rmcr.2014.09.004.

50. Colt HG, Crawford SW. In vitro study of the safety limits of bronchoscopic argon plasma coagulation in the presence of airway stents. Respirology 2006;11(5):643–7.

51. Plojoux J, Laroumagne S, Vandemoortele T, et al. Management of benign dynamic "a-shape" tracheal stenosis: A retrospective study of 60 patients. Ann Thorac Surg 2015;99(2):447–53.

9780443182747